WeightWatchers®

HEALTHY PARENT
Healthy Child

First published in Great Britain by Simon & Schuster UK Ltd,
2009
A CBS Company

Simon & Schuster UK Ltd
1st Floor, 222 Gray's Inn Road, London WC1X 8HB

1 3 5 7 9 10 8 6 4 2

Editorial Consultant: Francine Lawrence
Editor: Sharon Amos
Design: Meg Georgeson

Weight Watchers Publications Team:
Jane Griffiths, Eileen Thornton

Printed and bound in China

ISBN 978 0 74329 549 9

WeightWatchers®

HEALTHY PARENT
Healthy Child

simple rules for a healthy-weight home

Karen Miller-Kovach

SIMON &
SCHUSTER

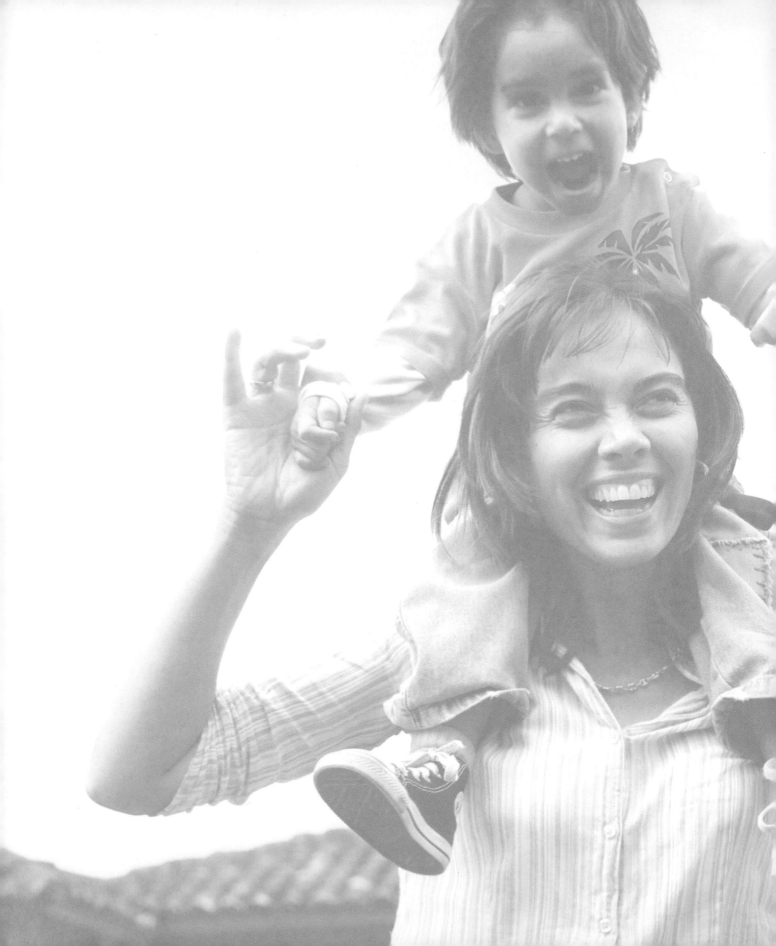

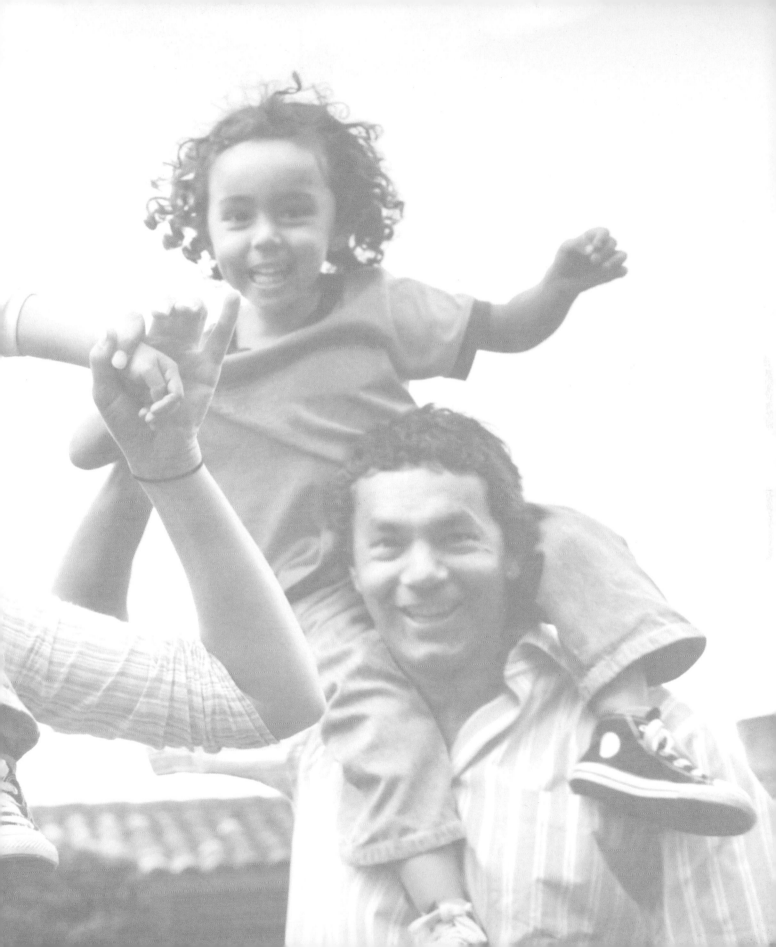

introduction

There is no question that the growing rate of excess weight among our children is an international concern and, as parents, we have the opportunity and the responsibility to make a real difference. That's what *Healthy Parent, Healthy Child* is all about.

Little did I know when I started working in this area several years ago that it would have a lasting impression on my life. I have never met a parent who didn't have the goal of raising healthy, happy children but I have met scores of parents who feel that they are somehow inadequate because their child or children are neither healthy nor happy because of their weight. It is not that these parents don't care. Indeed, they are among the most caring individuals I know. In some cases, they cared too much – but expressed that care in unhelpful ways like putting their child on structured diets or banning treats – so that the weight remained an issue and the dynamic of the family was impaired.

Healthy Parent, Healthy Child is a hands-on manual of the 'whys' and 'hows' to express your care as a parent in a positive, productive way. It is not a diet book (quite the opposite, in fact!) nor a rant against the fat-promoting society in which we live. Rather, it is a practical guide for all adults who have children in their care because it provides a way to instil habits that will last a lifetime.

It doesn't matter what the composition of your family is – whether you as parents have weight issues yourselves, whether you have children with weight issues, or a mixture of each – the rules of a healthy-weight home will benefit everyone. By teaching the basics of a healthy lifestyle and showing how everyday people (like you) have made them their family's way of life, you can make a difference. By living by the rules, you can not only improve your own, your partner's, and your children's weight, you can prevent the weight gain that is so common as we get older.

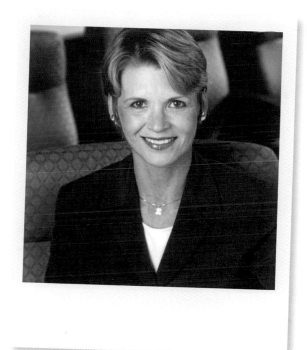

I am a scientist and it is scientific evidence that forms the basis of this book. I am also the mother of two fine young men. Growing up, one struggled with his weight while the other was very thin. As a single mum, I implemented what I was learning in my work life at home and did the best I could in creating a healthy-weight home. Despite the differences in my children's weight, the focus was the same – to eat wholesome foods, include treats and be active. Like many families, we struggled with limiting screen time.

I am happy to say that my sons are now independent adults and both are at a healthy weight; they eat well and are active. Most importantly, they look forward to having families of their own and raising their children in a healthy-weight home. I hope this book will help you to do that too.

Karen Miller-Kovach, M.S., R.D.
Chief Scientific Officer, Weight Watchers International

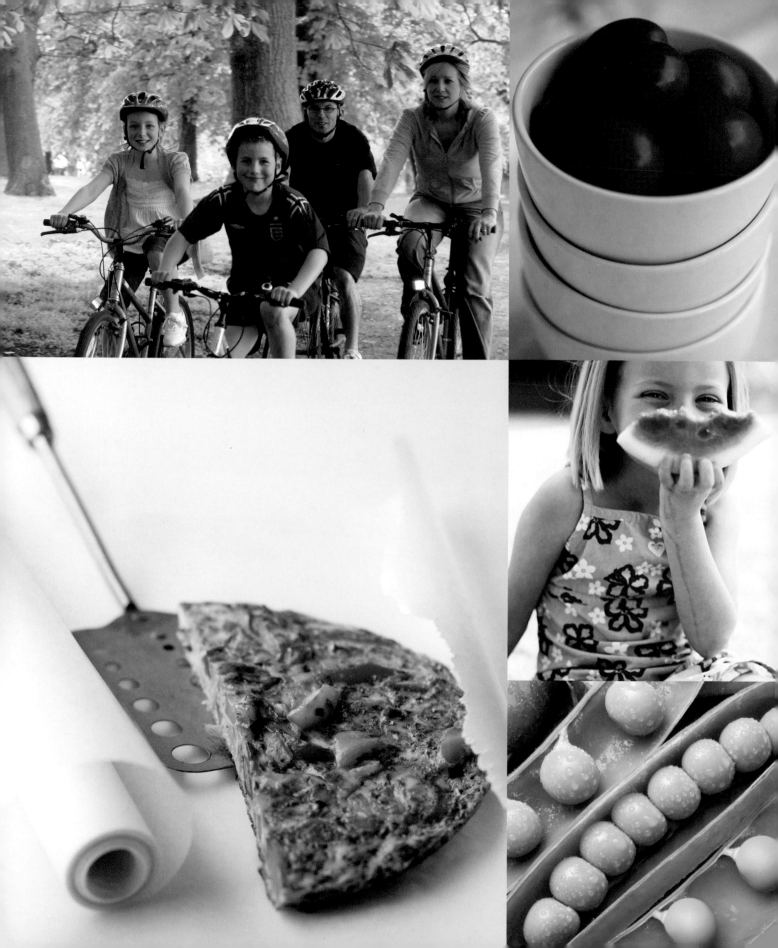

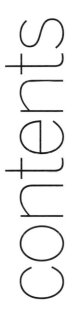

contents

part 1
the healthy
weight home

what is a healthy-weight home?

A healthy-weight home is one where every member of the household has a lifestyle that helps them to stay at a weight that is right and healthy for them – whether they tend to be heavier than average or thinner than usual.

The advice in this book will help you to create a healthy-weight home. It focuses on wholesome nutritious meals and snacks – including treats – combined with an active lifestyle plan to suit every member of the family.

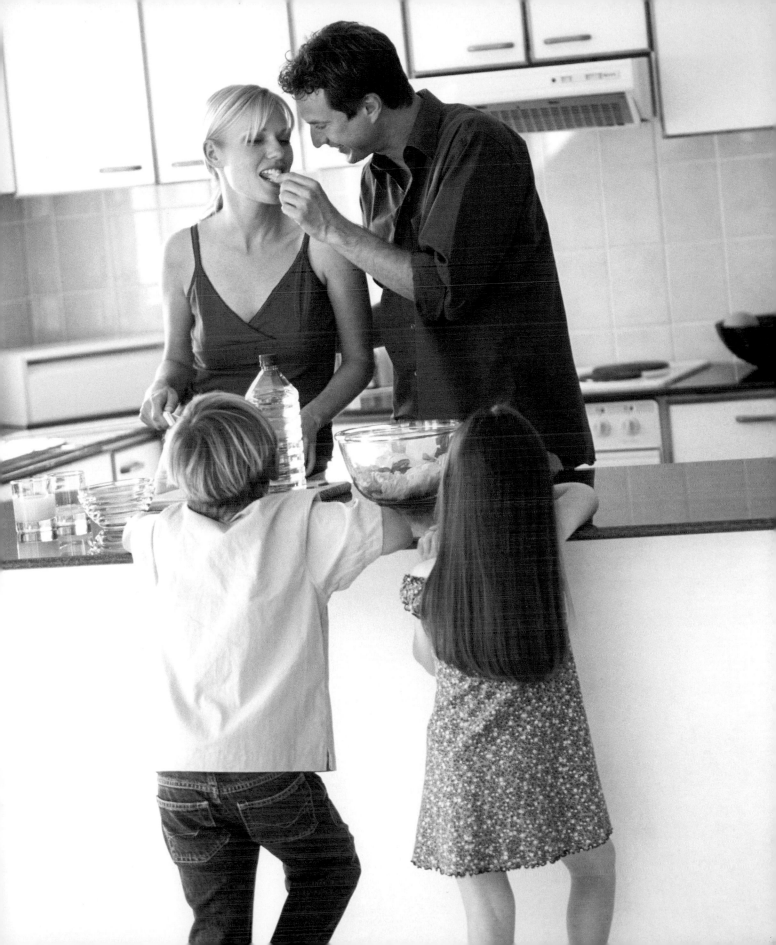

You are not alone

Now that you've decided to do something about your family's health, it's good to know that you don't have to go it alone. You probably know the kinds of changes you need to make to your lifestyle, but could do with some ideas and strategies to put them into practice. Many families are in exactly the same situation, where they need to take a fresh look at the way they live to help every member achieve and maintain a healthy weight. That's where this book will help you on each and every step of the way.

The advice in this book is good for all families, whether they include an overweight child or not, but if you do have a child who is overweight, it may be reassuring to know that it is a modern and increasingly common condition. To put the facts in perspective, a survey carried out for the Department of Health in 2000, found that 27% of girls in England aged between 2 and 19 years were overweight, and 7% were diagnosed as obese. The figures for boys were slightly lower at 20% overweight and 5% obese. (The word 'obese' is a medical term that is generally used when someone weighs more than 20% above the maximum weight for their height. For more information and charts see Chapter 4.)

Children who gain too much weight are more likely to develop weight-related illnesses such as diabetes while they are still young. They are also more likely to become overweight adults with all the associated risks of heart disease, arthritis, diabetes and other long-term health problems.

In fact, adult obesity rates have quadrupled in the UK over the past 25 years: 39% of the adult

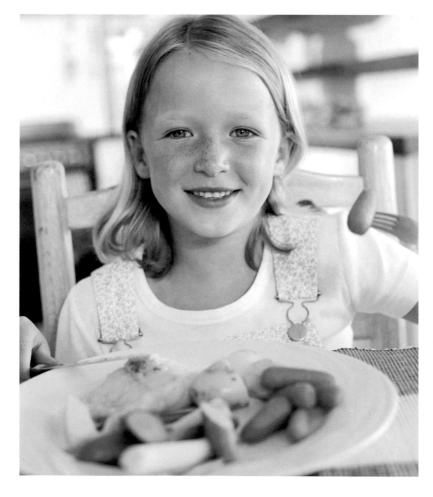

population are now overweight while 23% are actually obese. If these trends continue, the Royal College of Physicians has predicted that 33% of adults, 20% of boys and 33% of girls will be obese by 2020.

The problem of overweight children is not just a UK phenomenon: it's happening all over the world. In the US more than nine million children over the age of six are obese, and in Europe, Finland, Ireland and Greece have the highest rates of overweight 13-year-olds. Excess weight in children has even become an issue in countries where it has never been experienced before, such as China. In 2003, a study in Beijing found that 28% of boys and 14% of girls were significantly overweight.

This may sound depressing, but your family does not have to be part of these statistics. You have already taken the first step and with the help of this book you can make small changes to your lifestyle that will make a huge difference to your family's well-being and their future health.

Why is this happening?

Experts all over the world agree that the main reasons can be found in our own lifestyles, where:

- **processed foods are replacing wholesome less-processed foods**
- **fast food is widely available**
- **the need to be active as part of daily life is declining**

Understanding the reasons behind the trend is important, because they point us towards the solutions. There are many different ways that we can make a difference to our children's weight, and you

THE ADVICE YOU WILL FIND IN THIS BOOK IS GOOD FOR ALL FAMILIES EVERYWHERE – REGARDLESS OF WHETHER THEY INCLUDE AN OVERWEIGHT CHILD OR NOT

can create a strategy to suit your family's lifestyle.

Making science work for you

As the largest provider of weight-loss services in the world, Weight Watchers is concerned about the growing numbers of overweight children, and is absolutely committed to helping discover safe, lasting solutions.

Over the years, various scientific studies have made recommendations on tackling excess weight in childhood but it isn't always easy to translate these into everyday information that you can use at home. That's why Weight Watchers experts have taken this research and developed a programme that is scientifically sound, but also practical.

Healthy Parent, Healthy Child arms you with the latest scientific research that you can use to oversee the weight and health of your family, whether members are overweight, underweight or at

USE THE LATEST SCIENTIFIC RESEARCH TO OVERSEE THE WEIGHT AND HEALTH OF EVERYONE IN YOUR FAMILY

a healthy weight right now. (You'll find a complete list of scientific references at the end of the book.)

By following the Weight Watchers approach below, you'll be on your way to a healthy-weight home.

Why Weight Watchers?

Since 1963, Weight Watchers has helped millions of people all over the world lose weight.

With its science-based tactics and talent for translating medical recommendations into practical advice, Weight Watchers is uniquely qualified to tackle the problem and find weight-loss solutions for adults.

The Weight Watchers approach is based on four key ideas:

- making wise food choices
- being physically active
- developing positive thinking skills
- living in a supportive environment

While this method has been extensively tested on adults, it has not been looked at for children. Weight Watchers does not encourage children to join its traditional adult programme and no child under 10 can become a Weight Watchers member. In fact, no popular weight-loss methods have been tested on children.

So Weight Watchers took on the challenge of finding ways to help children become a healthy weight. The Chief Scientific Officer for Weight Watchers in the USA, Karen Miller-Kovach, a parent herself, developed a family-based pilot project to help parents make science-based recommendations – which have been proved to affect children's weight – part of their daily routine.

In addition to the pilots that have run in the USA and the UK, *Healthy Parent, Healthy Child* now makes the ideas from the family programme available to everyone and is the starting point for you to turn your household into a healthy-weight home.

Children have an inbuilt advantage

When it comes to weight loss, children have an energy advantage over adults. They are still growing (unless they are older teens) and that process uses up energy or calories all by itself. Children's

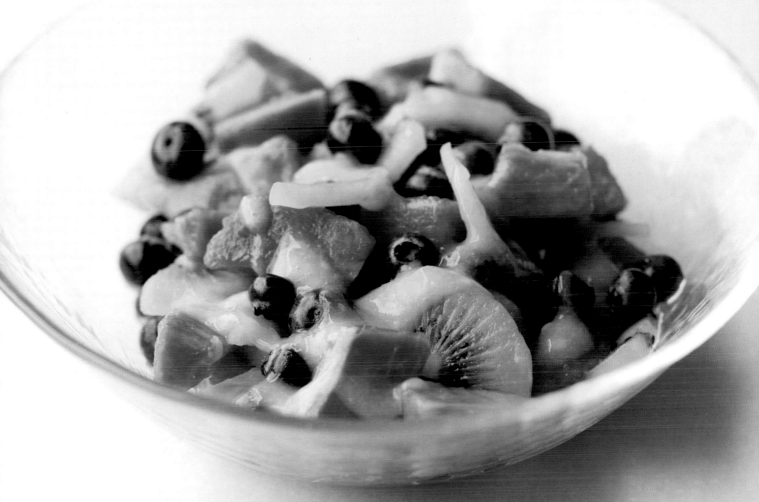

bodies also respond better than adults' when they increase their activity levels. These two factors combine to help them achieve and sustain a healthy weight with fewer restrictions on what they eat, compared to an adult aiming to lose weight.

Living in a healthy-weight home where all family members have a lifestyle that includes nutritious food and regular physical activity can make a big difference to children. It can stop and even reverse the pattern of weight gain that leads to obesity.

To create a healthy-weight home all you need to do is make small consistent changes in a few key areas rather than following a structured low-calorie diet and strict exercise programme. It's a realistic approach to reducing excess weight in children and enhancing the health of all members of the family. And that's just what you'll find in the pages of *Healthy Parent, Healthy Child.*

The book is a team effort that includes input from weight-loss experts, paediatricians, counsellors and – most importantly – families. In the book you'll find case studies of families who have turned their lives around thanks to Weight Watchers family-based approach.

how to be an effective parent

We parents are like the sun at the centre of the solar system and our children are planets in orbit around us. The sun's influence on the planets is enormous and so is the effect parents have on children. The most obvious examples are the way we shape our children's eating habits and how active they are. Our children's health is deeply affected by our own health, our relationships and parenting styles.

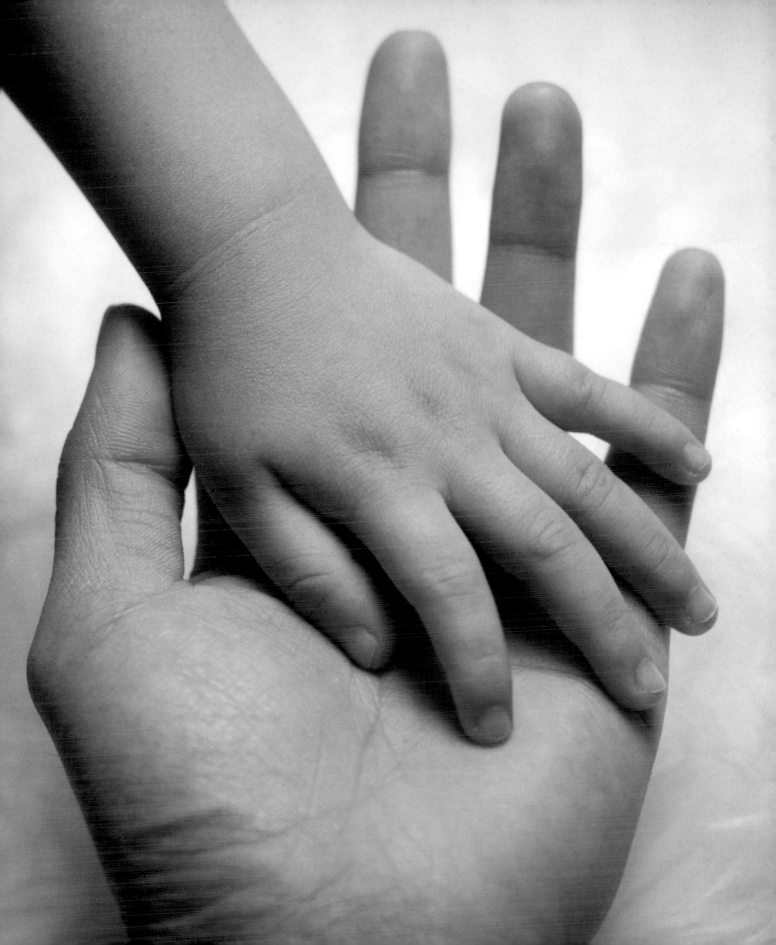

The roles parents play

Research on the role of parents in creating a healthy-weight home has been going on for more than 30 years all over the world. Results show that children who are most successful in managing their weight come from supportive families with good relationships between family members. Their parents also use strategies to give their children a positive self-image and a sense of responsibility.

As parents, we play five major roles in our children's lives.

1 We are **ROLE MODELS** who show our children how to eat well and have an active lifestyle by doing it ourselves.

2 We are **PROVIDERS** who put food on the table and buy our children toys and sports equipment that encourage activity.

3 We are **ENFORCERS** who set out the family's food and activity policies and then make sure that we follow them consistently.

4 We are **PROTECTORS** who look out for our children, both physically and emotionally.

5 We are **AGENTS FOR CHANGE** who spread the word about the benefits of a healthy-weight home.

As parents, we are responsible for creating a healthy-weight home and it is really important that we understand each of the five roles.

BEING A ROLE MODEL

We are the most significant role models our children will ever have and they will model themselves on our behaviour. But we are not the only ones. Research shows that in families with more than one child, older siblings can also be role models. Childminders, too, take on the role. That's why it's so important for everyone to work together and follow the same rules.

Being a role model is closely connected with just about every aspect of a child's behaviour, especially those that affect their weight. For example, toddlers who are fussy eaters tend to take after other family members who are also picky about food.

Role models have a big effect on activity. In one study of four to seven year olds, children with active mothers were twice as likely to be active themselves as those with mothers who were more sedentary. When fathers were included in the equation, children with active dads were three and a half times more likely to be active. And when both parents followed an active lifestyle their children were almost six times more likely to do so as well. The researchers believe that role modelling was a major influence on the children they studied. Children learn by what they see and the influence of a role model is crucial.

BEING A PROVIDER

As parents, our children depend on us to provide everything, from clothing and shelter to food. That's fine all the time the children are at home under our care, but what happens when they are looked after by someone else (see information panel below)? This is when food becomes a particular issue, especially for working parents who use childcare services to look after their children outside the home. In this case the nursery or childminder looking after your child takes on the role of provider.

In England childcare services and registered childminders must follow National Standards on food and drink set out by the Department for Children, Schools and Families. The National Standards simply state that children should be 'provided with regular drinks and food in adequate quantities for their needs'. They go on to say that food and drink should be 'properly prepared, nutritious and complies with dietary requirements' and also state that childminders should keep a record of a child's special dietary requirements, preferences or food allergies.

As these guidelines are very general – and they are only guidelines and not legally enforceable – the best way to keep an eye on what your child is eating is to talk directly to the childminder and tell them what you want them to give your child. But bear in mind that you may have to be flexible; it's not practical to expect a childminder looking after five children, for example, to prepare five different meals at lunchtime.

PARENTS OFTEN ASK

How can I tell my childminder what I want?

As a general rule, the direct approach is best. If you want your child to drink water at meal times, then say so. If you don't want your child to watch tv after school, you need to give specific instructions. Never assume your childminder knows what you want; you need to spell it out.

WHO LOOKS AFTER MY CHILDREN?

When we talk about childminders in this book, we aren't just referring to officially registered childminders, we mean everyone who looks after your children, from grandparents and babysitters to aunts and au pairs, neighbours and friends. For your plan to create a healthy-weight home to have the best chance of success, you need to get all of them involved and tell them exactly what you need them to do – from how much tv you want your child to watch to what you want them to eat for breakfast.

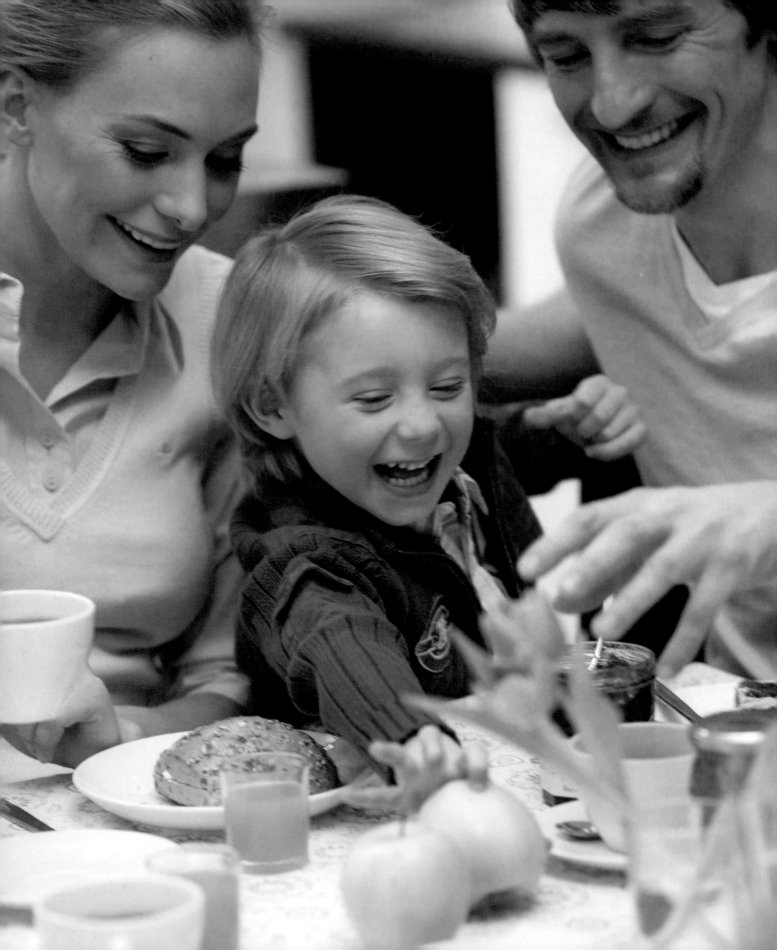

BEING AN ENFORCER

Families need structure to be able to follow household rules. The enforcer is the one who establishes the rules and helps family members follow them. Effective enforcers are not rigid and authoritarian, nor are they the 'food police'. Instead they decide how rules are put into effect and they apply the rules in a consistent way that supports healthy food choices, eating behaviours and leisure-time activities.

Enforcers need to be flexible. While children need structure, they also need rules that can be adapted. For example, an enforcer will realise that eating treats at a birthday party will probably balance out over a week of wholesome meals and snacks, and so won't try to stop their child enjoying party food.

Enforcers recognise that each member of the family is different. While everyone has to follow the same rules, the way in which each person follows them might not be the same. An older child may meet activity recommendations by taking up a team sport, while a toddler can be active just by playing in the garden with friends.

Research suggests that how stubborn a child is about following house rules stays relatively steady over time, with a peak in early adolescence and a decrease in the late teen years. Studies also show that children who resist rules are more likely to be aggressive and blame their problems on other people. Children who won't stick to house rules, like tidying up after themselves or coming home at a specific time, are also more likely to resist the rules for a healthy-weight home, which are set out in Chapter 6. And if they have weight problems, they are likely to blame these on other people.

Being consistent is the key to success. Inconsistent enforcing of family rules causes even more problems. All the adults in the house must be in agreement on sticking to rules and on how to deal with a child who steps out of line.

Finding the right approach

Research shows that children do best when their parents adapt their parenting skills to fit a child's nature, personality and needs.

Children need unconditional love and quality time. Authoritative parenting that balances affection with consistent boundaries increases the likelihood of raising happy, cooperative and confident children. Rigidly authoritarian parents and permissive parents tend to be less successful.

Experts agree it is better to guide children in the right direction rather

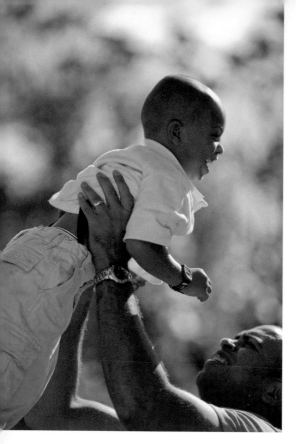

TAKING STEPS TO PROTECT OUR CHILDREN'S HEALTH NOW CAN HAVE A POSITIVE EFFECT THAT LASTS INTO ADULTHOOD

than dictate to them. Guiding food choices helps children to make their own decisions rather than simply learn that some foods are ok and others are not.

Similarly, with encouragement, a child's interest in exercise can be sparked by getting them to try different activities, by supporting them in their choice and by showing confidence in their abilities. For example, you might try going swimming once a week or get the children to choose a kite and then take them to a local beauty spot to fly it. Go out for the day: plan a bike ride to a fun destination and take a picnic with you. Take the children to see a musical to inspire them, then enrol them in a dance class. Or what about a martial arts class? You could buy everyone a pedometer and see how many miles the family can clock up in a week.

BEING A PROTECTOR

In today's world, the role of protecting our children has shifted from physical issues such as discipline in schools to emotional issues like bullying and feelings of isolation. The role of protector

extends outside the family: schools and the government are involved too. Research has shown that taking steps to protect our children's health now can have a positive effect that lasts into adulthood. Ways you can do this include supporting your children at home, making sure they have a safe environment to play in or walk to school in, and limiting their exposure to advertising for junk food targeted at children.

Children who feel secure in the protection of an adult will learn how to explore their surroundings in a safe and positive way.

BEING AN AGENT FOR CHANGE

As agents for change we can help create a healthy-weight environment for our children outside the home too. With their parents around to guide them, children can make healthy food choices and keep active at home. But what happens when they are at school, for example?

Children can't be expected to follow family food rules on their own. And they're rarely in a position to argue for changes to the menu or the school curriculum. This is where parents can get involved and act as agents for change.

It's often easier to change things if a group of people get together. In the seaside town of Deal in Kent, for example, when the school meals contract came up for tender, a group of parents, school governors and local business people formed a company, Whole School Meals, and successfully bid to take on the service. Now they cater for more than 20 local schools, providing freshly cooked meals using local seasonal produce. (See Chapter 11 for the full story.)

On a different tack, parents with a passion for sport can help run inspirational after-school clubs to add to the range of activities on offer at school. Enthusiastic football or cricket coaches are welcomed with open arms at most primary schools.

PARENTS NEED TO BE PARENTS

Children thrive on structure. They look to us to set the rules and enforce them – everything from getting them to brush their teeth to telling them when to be home for tea. In creating a healthy-weight home, structure comes from the parenting roles described in this chapter and from using them to make a set of family rules part of everyday life. We'll be coming to the rules themselves in Chapter 6, but examples include providing your children with a limited supply of treats or aiming to spend more time outdoors as a family. Over the weeks and years the rules will need to evolve as the children grow up.

As parents we have the power to change our family's attitudes to health and weight. We are in the best position to shift the family's worries from losing weight to focusing on living a healthy lifestyle. But responsibility has to be shared by everyone, including all family members and childminders. Managing weight is not something that anyone can do on their own.

Functioning as a family

A child's ability to assess and handle the relationships that are part of everyday life is affected by how well his or her family functions. Research shows that family togetherness makes a big difference. Members of families that function well feel connected to each other – children feel close to their parents and to each other. Families are dynamic: parents influence the children and each other, while children force their parents to change and adjust as they grow. Family solidarity is a powerful factor in changing habits.

the difference between adults and children

If our body weight is the result of a combination of what we eat and how active we are, then surely following a weight-loss diet should work equally well for children and adults? For years that's what many experts assumed – and some still do. But the reality is a lot more complicated. Children are not mini adults and their energy requirements are very different. Children are growing all the time and it is impossible to work out an average daily calorie intake for a child in the same way that you can for an adult. The key to managing a child's weight lies in a family-based approach and creating a healthy-weight home.

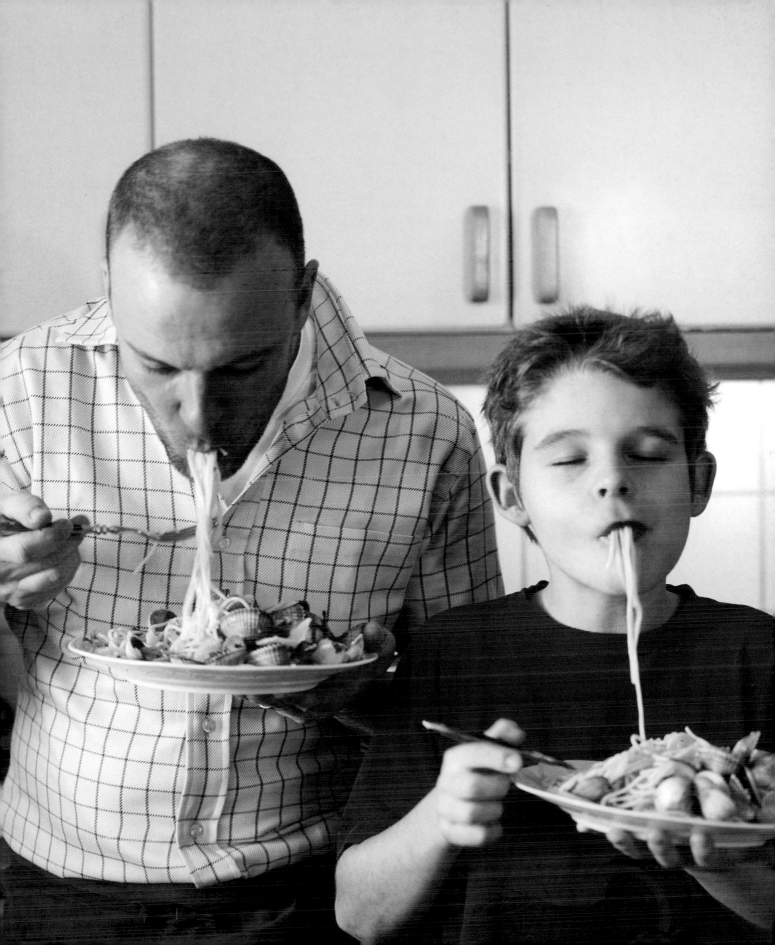

Why don't adult weight-loss programmes work for most children?

Mainly because adult programmes are too structured and don't include enough family involvement. Asking a child to follow a strict diet and exercise plan can make them dig their heels in, as well as causing conflict at home when they are the only one being singled out in this way. A family-based approach that is not overly strict and done with a lot of support makes much more sense.

Getting the energy balance right

One thing that children and adults have in common is the law of thermodynamics. This states that a person's weight is the result of the number of calories they eat and the amount of calories they use up. In other words, our weight is controlled by the number of calories 'in' and the number of calories 'out'.

If a child takes in more calories than they need for their current rate of growth and level of activity, then they will gain weight. Conversely, a child who is not taking in enough calories to 'fuel' growth and activity will lose weight. In children this process is often referred to as 'growing into their weight.'

Changes to either side of the equation will affect a child's weight. In a healthy-weight home, the calories 'in' side of the equation can be reduced by focusing on foods and drinks that are lower in calories but high in nutrients. These are known as low-energy density, high-nutrient density foods and drinks. The calories 'out' side of the equation has two elements. The first is physical activity, which burns up energy or calories. The second is time spent in sedentary activities that do not use up many calories – such as watching tv or playing computer games. The two

elements are closely linked, as reducing the amount of time spent sitting around frees up time for physical activity.

What about genes?

All biological families share a common gene pool. There is no doubt that children are more likely to gain excess weight in a family where some members are already overweight. But we also know that genes can't be blamed for today's increase in the number of overweight children. Genetic changes take many generations to develop – they don't appear over

WE CAN'T BLAME GENES FOR TODAY'S INCREASE IN THE NUMBER OF OVERWEIGHT CHILDREN

the course of a few decades. Luckily there is a big difference between being at risk of becoming overweight and actually doing so. Biology is not destiny. Several studies have shown that it is not uncommon for overweight children to become adults with a healthy weight. In one study 31% of obese children went on to become adults with a normal weight. Conversely, being a thin child does not protect you from gaining weight in later life.

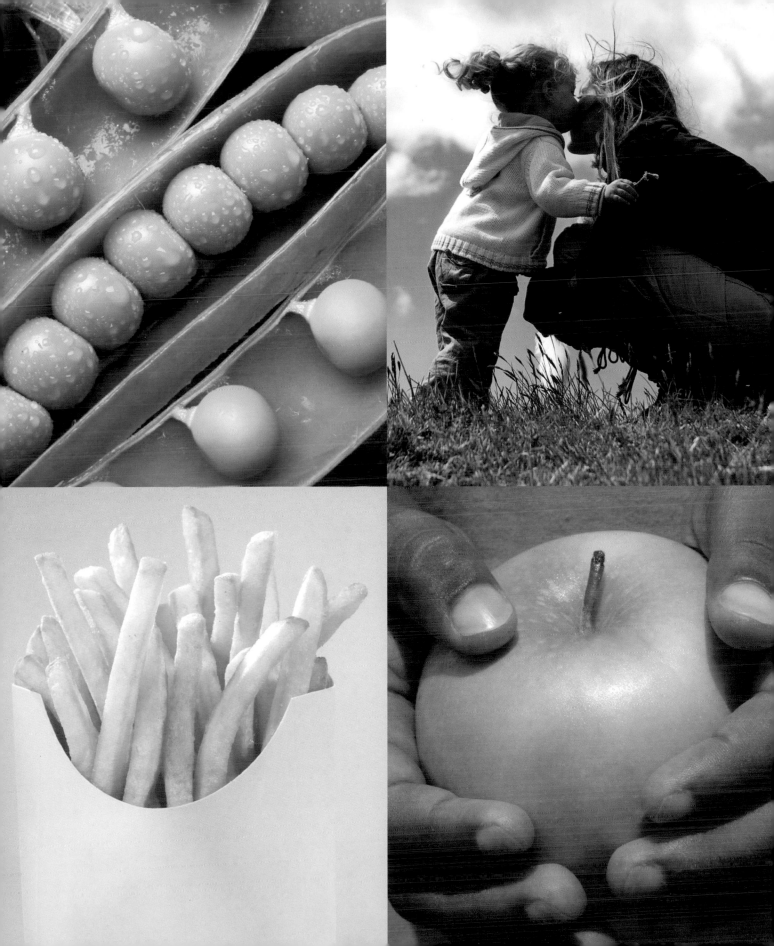

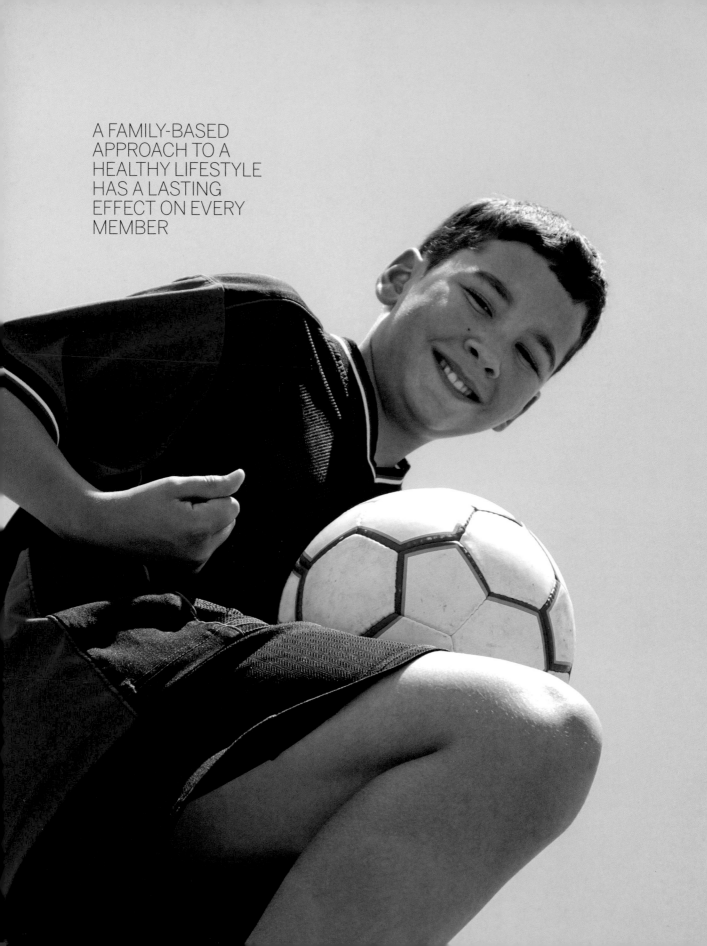

A FAMILY-BASED
APPROACH TO A
HEALTHY LIFESTYLE
HAS A LASTING
EFFECT ON EVERY
MEMBER

In the same study a further 30% of slim children became obese adults. A family-based approach to a healthy lifestyle has been shown to have a lasting effect on the whole family, despite any genetic tendency to excess weight.

I haven't got time

Changing behaviour takes time. In one family-based weight programme, participants said that lack of time was the main reason for not following the exercise and eating plans. The same complaint came up in a study that looked at adolescents. The teenage girls who did not lead an active lifestyle said it was because they didn't have time. But it really is possible to make progress towards a healthy-weight home in a normal daily timetable.

PARENTS OFTEN ASK

Why does one of my children have a weight problem while the others do not?

There is no simple answer. While families share a common gene pool, each individual has a different mix, so some children may be more prone to gaining weight than others. This tendency may not become apparent until a child is older. Children have different personalities too, which can influence weight-related behaviour.

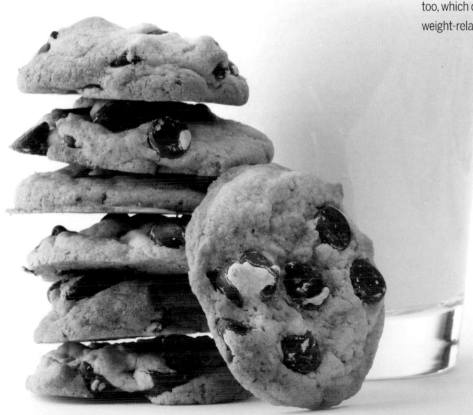

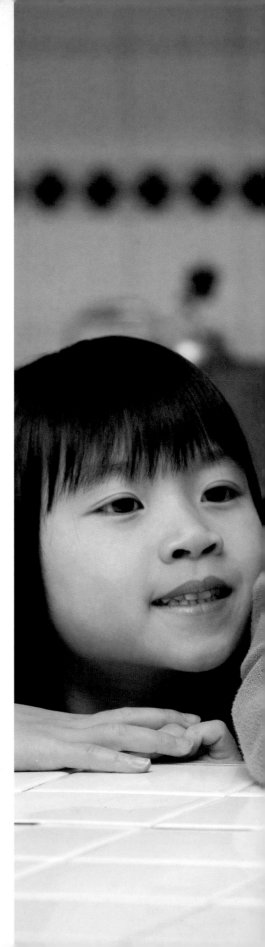

If my child has a weight problem but I don't, why do I have to change my behaviour?
As a parent you are the biggest influence on your child's life. Being a role model and making changes along with your child shows support and family solidarity – and that makes all the difference. Plus you'll be improving your own health at the same time – so everyone benefits.

It's just a matter of choosing carefully which changes you are going to make to your lifestyle and then sticking to them consistently.

Children need extra calories

Although weight is all about a balance between calories 'in' and calories 'out', the equation doesn't work in quite the same way for children as for adults. Children need extra calories for growth and development. Children who eat about the right amount of calories that they need for growth, daily metabolism and physical activity gain weight at a pace that is in line with their increasing height.

Children who eat more calories than they require will gain more weight than they need to compensate for their increase in height. Those who eat less become thinner in relation to their height. In extreme cases where a child is not getting enough calories, their height may even be restricted.

Both adults and children with weight problems are eating more calories than their bodies need, but a typical child's diet differs from an adult's. In many western countries a typical child's diet is high in fat. Each teaspoon of fat contains 170-188 calories, compared to a teaspoon of pure protein or carbohydrate, which has about 85 calories. Chips, burgers,

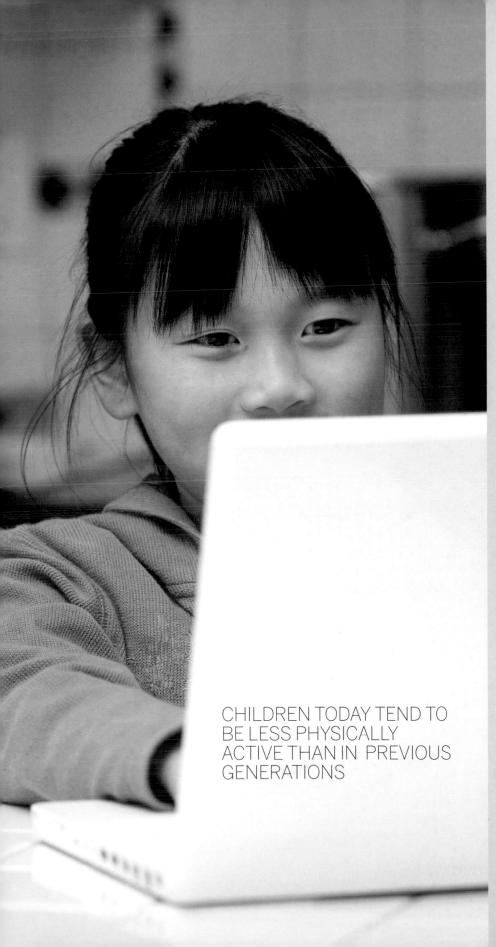

CHILDREN TODAY TEND TO BE LESS PHYSICALLY ACTIVE THAN IN PREVIOUS GENERATIONS

PARENTS OFTEN ASK

What should I do if my child starts worrying about their weight?

The best approach is to shift the focus from their weight to being healthy. Weight management is, after all, about healthy living. Point out the advantages of a healthy lifestyle – clear skin and shiny hair, not getting out of breath during PE or football, waking up full of energy in the mornings. Focusing on these positive changes will help each member of the family achieve a healthy weight at the same time.

chicken nuggets and biscuits are a few of the high-fat foods in a typical child's diet. Most children also get extra calories from foods that are high in calories compared to their nutritional value – such as soft drinks (including fruit juice) and so-called snack foods.

Children and activity

Activity patterns in children and adults are quite different. Adults tend to be more sedentary and even children today tend to be less

LACK OF ACTIVITY IS CLOSELY RELATED TO THE AMOUNT OF TIME SPENT WATCHING TV OR PLAYING COMPUTER GAMES

active than in previous generations. Lack of activity is closely related to the amount of time we spend watching tv, surfing the net or playing computer games. This double whammy of more calories 'in' and fewer 'out' is at the root of the rapid rise in children's weight.

But the biggest difference between children and adults lies in home life. One of the greatest advances has been to acknowledge the influence that parents have on their children – and that's something we can use to our advantage.

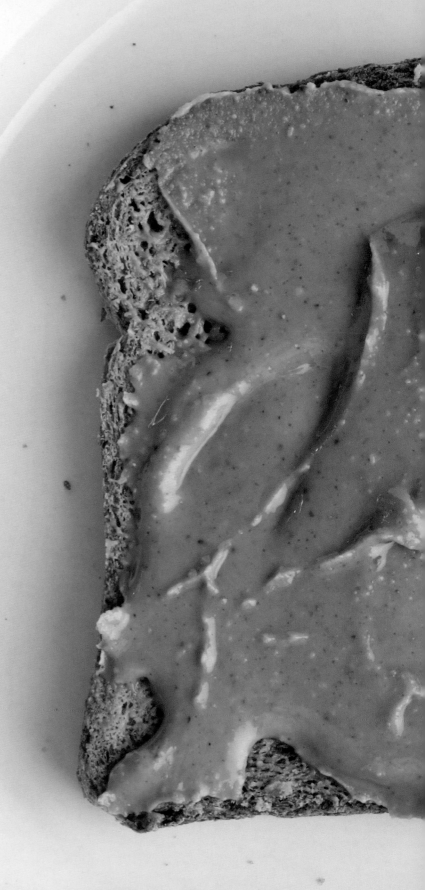

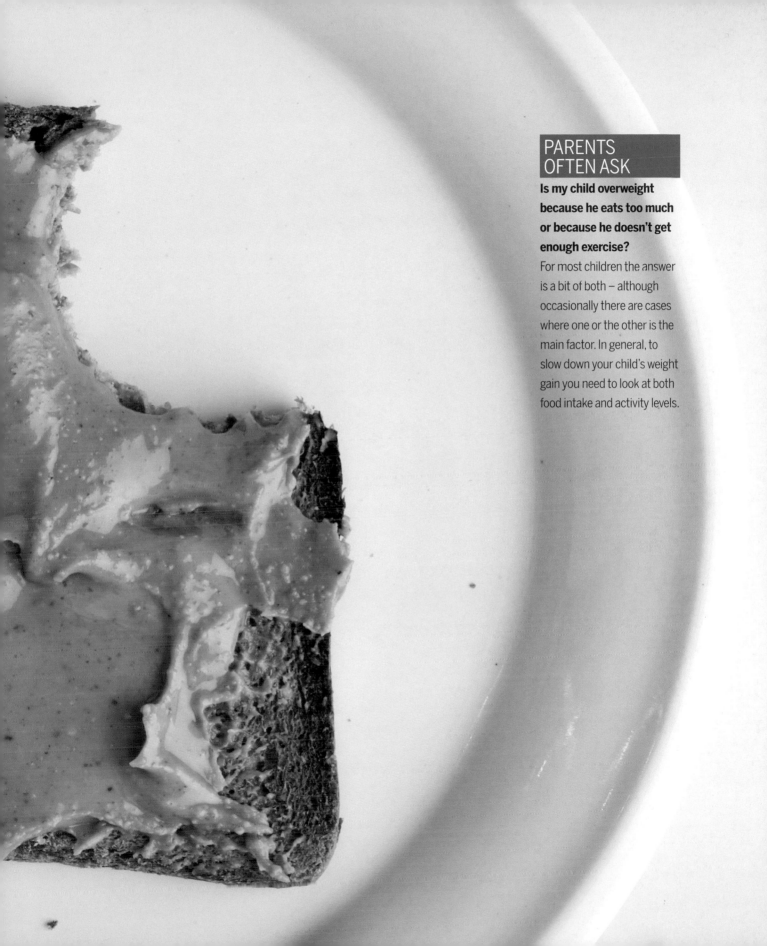

PARENTS OFTEN ASK

Is my child overweight because he eats too much or because he doesn't get enough exercise?

For most children the answer is a bit of both – although occasionally there are cases where one or the other is the main factor. In general, to slow down your child's weight gain you need to look at both food intake and activity levels.

case study 1

Rachel Fryer and her husband Andy wanted to be healthier and they wanted their two-year-old son Harry to have the best start in life. Creating a healthy-weight home brings together all the changes they need to make to their lifestyle and gives Harry a great foundation to build on

I am determined that Harry will grow up with a healthy attitude towards food. I don't want him to see food as an issue, as I did when I was a child, when I wasn't allowed to leave the table until I'd finished. And I want him to be healthier than I was when I was growing up.

When I decided that my family was going to live in a healthy-weight home, the first thing I focused on was eating together as often as possible. It's difficult as I am a Weight Watchers leader, running six meetings a week, and Andy does shift work so his hours constantly vary. Even Harry is out at nursery all day Thursday and Friday.

The one time when we are often together is breakfast. And one of the first things I had to do was persuade Andy to eat anything at all. He'd always say he didn't want breakfast, then he'd be making himself a snack before it was even 10am. I asked him to start trying for Harry's sake. I said, if he sees you having a snack he'll want one too.

I shop better than I used to because I plan everything. I do an internet shop with a week's menus in mind. Then, say the night before, I decide, right, we'll have beef stroganoff tomorrow. I like to stay one step ahead. It takes the pressure off. Otherwise I waste time thinking about what to cook. And by structuring the week's menus, it frees me up to do things that I enjoy,

like swimming or going for a run by myself.

Andy's favourite activity is to go off on his bike – he's been threatening to get me one with a seat on the back so that Harry can come too but I'm a bit nervous. Instead, I prefer it when we all go to the beach together for a game of football.

We're still cutting down on tv. I realised it wasn't Harry who put the tv on, it was me. I've made a conscious effort not to do that any more.

Although Harry is only two, I'm committed to letting him serve himself at meal times. If I put the food on his plate, he eats selectively. But the more he sees others helping themselves, the more he'll follow suit. It's not easy: there's more preparation and more washing up with all the serving bowls. But even when we're just having a sandwich at lunch time I set out bowls of grapes or carrot sticks for Harry to help himself. At dinner it can get messy. At first Harry put about 400 peas on his plate, then didn't eat a single one.

At the beginning it was a major problem going to visit family and friends. The first thing my parents would say when we walked through the door was, 'Harry, would you like a chocolate?' But now I've explained to them all about creating a healthy-weight home, they are very supportive.

Of course, like any small child, Harry still asks for a

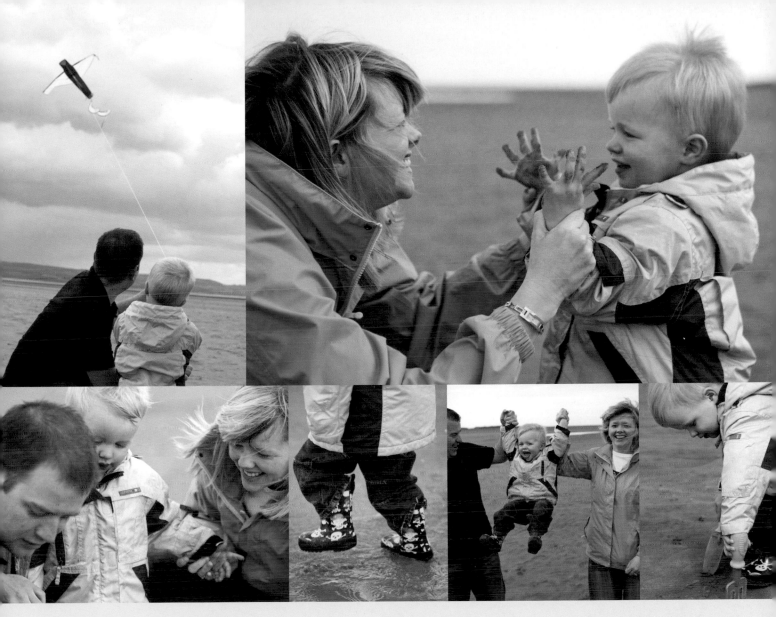

biscuit when he's hungry but I have strategies ready. I say, 'Would you like an apple or a pear, or a yoghurt?' and mostly he takes me up on that. But if it's really close to meal time I try to distract him instead and say, 'Come and help mummy set the table.'

As an agent for change I like to spread the word to friends and show them that these methods really work. When we had tea at the play centre I persuaded the other mums that we should put out snacks in bowls and let the kids help themselves. Once they stopped worrying about the mess, they could see

LIVING IN A HEALTHY-WEIGHT HOME GIVES YOU THE CONFIDENCE TO CAMPAIGN FOR CHANGE

what a good idea it was.

I also talked to Harry's nursery as I had a few issues with their menu, which featured foods like chicken nuggets, fish fingers and potato shapes. It turned out some other mums felt the same way too and after discussion with the nursery the children can now choose from a healthier menu, with options such as wholemeal wraps, vegetable pizzas, and fruit and veg snacks. It's the perfect example of how being committed to a healthy-weight home gives you the confidence to campaign for change.

understanding your child's weight

Appearances can be deceptive when trying to assess your child's weight. There are plenty of other factors to take into account besides actual body weight, including age, height, and whether they are going through a growing spurt. Here's some of the science behind looking at children's weight.

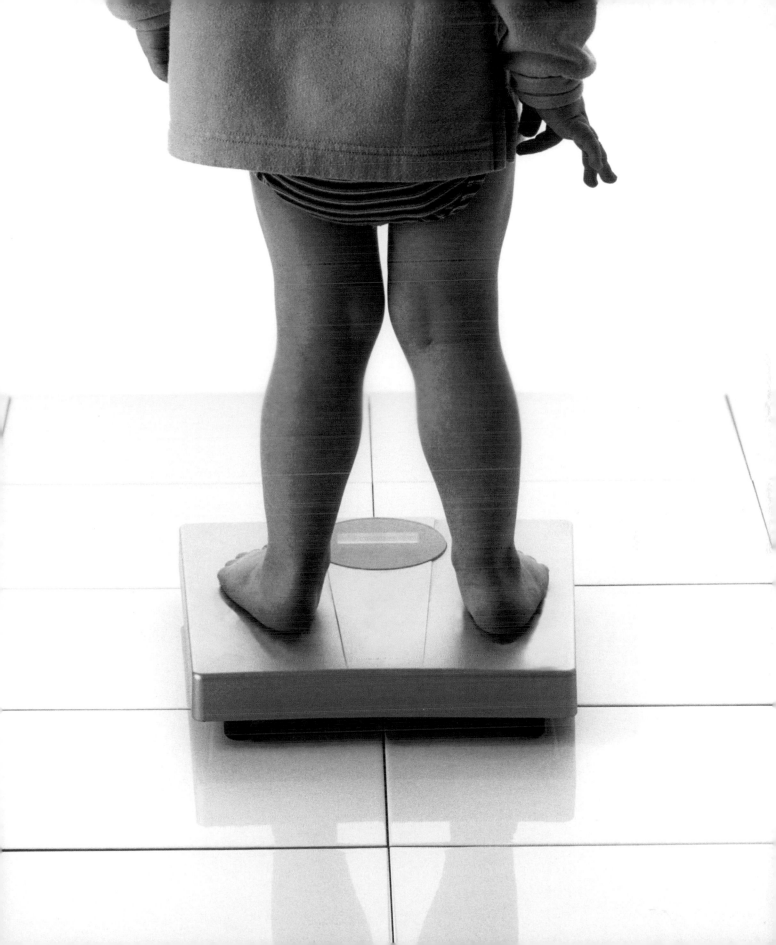

What is Body Mass Index?

Researchers around the world need technical definitions so that they can compare the results of their studies. To evaluate research into weight they use a system called the Body Mass Index or BMI. BMI is used for both adults and children, and for most people it gives an accurate indication of the amount of fat on the body. You can calculate your own BMI by dividing your weight in kilograms by your height in metres squared.

If this sounds too complicated, various health websites with online calculators will do the maths for you. Go to the NHS website www.nhsdirect.nhs.uk/ then click on *Mind and Body Magazine* and again on Interactive Tools. Then input your height and weight (use metric or imperial measurements) into the BMI calculator and it will work it out for you. It's surprisingly easy to do. A child's BMI is calculated in exactly the same way.

By checking a BMI against a specific chart (see opposite) you can find out whether your child is at risk of becoming overweight or is actually already overweight. Charts to check a child's BMI are based on their age because BMIs change depending on the child's development. And because boys and girls grow at different rates, separate charts are used for each.

These BMI-for-age charts are a more accurate way to assess a child's weight than just using body weight itself. They usually give a good indication of body-fat levels: a child who scores a high BMI-for-age number usually has a lot of body fat.

Paediatricians use BMI-for-age measurements to track a child's body size from childhood through adolescence and into adulthood. BMI charts for adults are the same for men and women, with the same ranges and cut-off points. For adults, a BMI of 19 or under is considered underweight; a BMI of 19 to 24.9 is a healthy weight; between 25 and 29.9 is overweight; while a BMI of 30 or above is obese.

BMI changes as a child grows

One of your first steps if you are worried about your child's weight is to see your family GP. He or she will use a BMI-for-age chart for reference, as appearances can be deceiving when assessing a child's weight – it's quite common for a chubby-looking toddler to have a BMI within the healthy weight range. By filling out a BMI-for-age graph at regular intervals your GP will be able to differentiate between normal weight gain for growth and excess weight gain.

BMI, body shape and body size change throughout childhood. As a

Should I weigh my child and, if so, how often?

It's generally not a good idea to weigh children because it gives them the message that weight is very important. It's better to leave weighing to routine school and health checks or to your GP if your child is under their care for weight-related health reasons. If you want to keep an eye on things at home, the way children's clothes are fitting will give you a good idea of what's going on.

Work out your child's BMI with the formula BMI = weight in kilos divided by height in metres squared (or use an online calculator); then use the charts below to check whether you need to take action

use this chart for boys

age	at risk of overweight if BMI is greater than	overweight if BMI is greater than
2 years	18.2	19.3
5 years	16.8	17.9
8 years	18.7	21.2
13 years	23	27
18 years	26.9	30.6

use this chart for girls

age	at risk of overweight if BMI is greater than	overweight if BMI is greater than
2 years	18	19.1
5 years	16.8	18.3
8 years	18.3	20.7
13 years	23.8	28.3
18 years	27.3	33.1

DEFINITIONS

'Overweight' is the term used for children with a very high BMI for their age. Adults with a comparable BMI would be defined as 'obese'.
'At risk of overweight' is the term used for children whose BMI is between the healthy and overweight limit. Adults with a comparable BMI are classified as 'overweight'.
In this book the terms 'obese' and 'obesity' are used to refer to the medical issues of excess weight in children and adults; they are not used to classify children's weight.

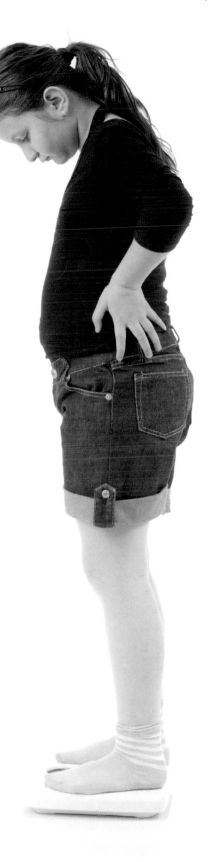

PARENTS
OFTEN ASK

My daughter is overweight. What sort of help can I expect from my GP?

All practices vary but your GP should be able to help you access the most appropriate help. For example, the surgery can help you monitor your daughter's weight by regularly weighing and measuring height to calculate her BMI – this might be done by the practice nurse for school-age children; the health visitor usually looks after young children. Your GP can refer you to a dietician for advice or they may suggest your daughter sees the school nurse if the dietician has a long waiting list. Doctors can also offer exercise on prescription, such as discounted sessions at the local swimming pool or gym. It's in your GP's interest to help you and your family be as healthy as possible.

child moves from being a toddler to preschool age, BMI typically drops, and growth slows to just over a kilo of weight for every 2.5cm increase in height. After the preschool years, BMI gradually increases.

From late primary school and into the beginning of puberty, children's bodies can look very different from each other. Some children grow much faster than others and body shapes change. Some children gain body fat before they grow taller as their body is storing fat ready for the growth spurt that goes with puberty.

During puberty boys' and girls' bodies change in different ways. A boy's body adds muscle and usually loses body fat, but boys develop more fat across the stomach. A girl adds both muscle and body fat, with fat going to breasts, hips and buttocks. Girls are more likely than boys to gain excess weight in adolescence.

The links between childhood BMI and overweight adults

Children with a high BMI-for-age are more likely to become obese adults. And the longer a child is overweight, the more likely it is that they will have weight problems as an adult. About a third of preschool children who are overweight become obese adults, rising to about half of overweight school-age children becoming obese adults. Children with a high BMI are twice as likely to become obese adults compared with children whose BMI is in the healthy weight range. The risk is greatest for children who have the highest BMI and who maintain a high BMI as they get older.

Children who carry excess weight into adulthood are also more likely to have weight-related illnesses, including heart disease and diabetes. The bottom line is to prevent excess weight gain at any early age. Bringing a high BMI down into the healthy range is important. Beyond health implications, being an overweight teen can have social issues, such as feeling isolated or being bullied.

Although these are sobering facts, there's no need to feel discouraged. Children have an enormous advantage over adults when it comes to managing their weight. They need more calories as they grow, so it is much simpler to make small changes in eating and activity patterns that can have a big impact on body weight.

When do children need to lose weight?

As a parent your first goal is to make sure that your child grows and develops normally. Your second goal is to help your child

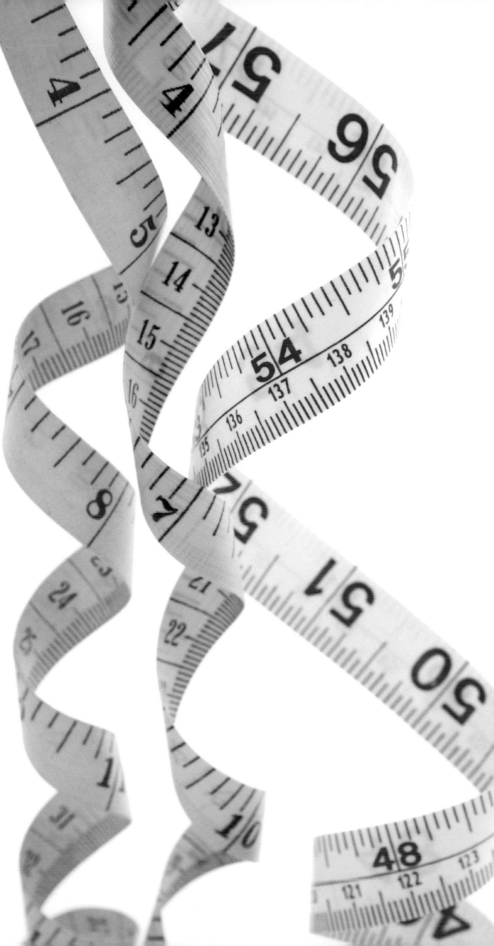

PARENTS OFTEN ASK

How can I tell if my child is overweight?

It is very difficult to look at a child and tell if he or she is overweight. As children grow and develop, their body shape changes. The only accurate way to tell is to calculate your child's BMI and plot the information on a BMI-for-age graph – your GP will do this for you.

My daughter is really thin. Does that mean she is anorexic?

Not necessarily. Anorexia nervosa is a medically diagnosed eating disorder that has several other characteristics besides low weight. Sufferers may starve themselves or make themselves sick after eating; they may exercise to extremes; they may have rituals about eating and they often picture themselves as being fat, even when they are not. If you have any concerns about a daughter or son – the disorder affects boys and girls – get in touch with your GP, who will be able to refer you to specialist help if necessary. (See also Chapter 13)

PARENTS OFTEN ASK

If my son is already overweight, does that mean that he will automatically become an obese adult?

While overweight children do have an increased risk of becoming overweight adults, it's not true of everyone – and it's easy to break the cycle. Half of all school-age children who are overweight go on to become adults with a healthy weight. Children who are already overweight will benefit from living in a healthy-weight home.

gradually reach a healthy weight.

Experts agree that it is best to start early. One strategy for young children is to slow down the rate at which they are gaining weight, so that their BMI-for-age does not keep going up. For example, a goal for very young children – two to four years old – whose BMI-for-age is near the top of the range might be to limit weight gain to less than one kilo for every 2.5cm increase in height.

Another strategy that's often recommended is to temporarily maintain your child at the same weight while they are growing. Then, as he or she gets taller, their BMI-for-age will automatically drop into the healthy-weight range. This approach is often used for children age four and over, who do not have weight-related health problems.

It is very rare for healthcare professionals to recommend that a child under the age of seven

actually needs to lose weight. The exception would be where a child with a BMI-for-age in the overweight range already has a weight-related medical condition such as high blood pressure or high blood cholesterol level.

The recommendations are similar for older children (aged seven and over). The goal for children whose BMI-for-age puts them in the overweight range is to maintain a steady weight as they grow taller. But children who are over seven, have a high BMI and weight-related medical problems, may be encouraged to lose weight.

Helping children to lose weight

Adult weight-loss programmes are not suitable for children. The only exception is for older teenagers who have reached their adult height and have a BMI of at least 30.

DOES MY CHILD NEED TO LOSE WEIGHT?

age	range of BMI for age	weight-related health problems?	treatment
Up to 7 years	At risk of overweight or overweight	No	Weight maintenance
Up to 7 years	Overweight	Yes	Consider weight loss
7 years and over	At risk of overweight	No	Weight maintenance
7 years and over	At risk of overweight or overweight	Yes	Weight loss
Late teens	BMI of at least 30	Yes or No	Weight loss on an adult programme

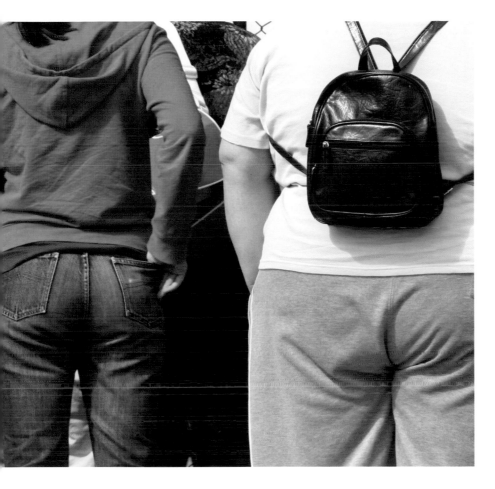

Weight-loss recommendations should be based on a child's age, how overweight they are and whether they have any weight-related health problems. Even when weight loss is recommended it should be done in a slow and gradual way. Current advice is that children should not be losing more than an average of half a kilo a month – unless they are under direct supervision by a paediatrician or doctor with experience in weight management.

Small weight changes can add up over the course of a year – half a kilo a month is six kilos a year. Add a couple of centimetres of growth and it is likely that a child's BMI-for-age will drop even lower. Slow weight loss lets a child grow taller at a normal rate and helps maintain muscle mass. Gradual loss is an achievable realistic goal. And the eating patterns that encourage slow weight loss are easier to stick to, as well as promoting normal growth and development.

PARENTS OFTEN ASK

Why is the recommended rate of weight loss so much lower for children than adults?

There is a big difference between the recommended half a kilo a month for children and half to one kilo a week for adults. First, children have much higher nutritional requirements than adults and so they need to eat a fair amount of food and calories. To lose weight more rapidly, a child would have to make big changes in lifestyle and eating habits, which can only be done by following a highly structured weight programme, and this type of approach usually backfires with children. Also, the slower weight is lost, the more likely it is to stay off, permanently.

case study 2

Michelle Ashwell has always struggled with her weight and has lost 3½ stone three times: this time she is determined to keep it off. By creating a healthy-weight home she knows she is giving herself and her family – husband Mark and children Dominic, 8, and Megan, 12 – the best chance. And she's been at her ideal weight for more than five years now

I've always battled with my weight and I think my son has the potential to have weight problems too. I want to keep my children out of that yo-yo cycle of gaining and losing pounds.

Like many families, we've found limiting screen time one of the toughest challenges. But in a healthy-weight home you're looking for progress, not perfection. My strategies for controlling how much tv we all watch include having only one tv and that's in the living room. We've also only got one family computer. And the Nintendo Wii games console is great – it gets the children up and moving, playing tennis for example, instead of being hunched over a games controller.

The children are now quite good at saving up viewing time to watch their favourite programmes, but in the early days there was a bit of confusion. Dominic came home from school one day and told me they'd watched a video about the ancient Egyptians in history. He said: 'But I didn't watch it, mummy, because I didn't want to waste my viewing time, so I looked out of the window.' I had to explain to him that programmes you watch at school don't count and neither do IT lessons. Children take things very literally.

To tempt the children away from the tv we've got a 12-foot trampoline in the garden that we all go on. Megan likes it when we have trampolining competitions – she says it's very funny when mummy and daddy do straddle jumps.

On Saturday mornings Megan does ballet, modern jazz and tap dancing in town with her friends. She walks to school every morning – it's about a mile – and walks to meet me after work three days a week – I'm a specialist nurse at the local hospital.

Megan and I also did the Race for Life together last year, running and jogging the five-kilometre course. Dominic enjoys football and he trains every Saturday morning and plays a match every Sunday.

We've got a fantastic activity role model in my husband Mark, who is an Iron Man Triathlete – that's swimming, cycling and running all in one event – and he has represented England in the European Long Course Triathlon Championship. He's also run 16 London Marathons. In the past it tended to be him who took the children to the park while I cooked supper or had an hour's peace and quiet, but now the family is following the 5 Simple Rules I know I have to join in too.

I've always gone for wholesome home-cooked meals so I was confident that the family was eating nutritious food, but I realised I needed to tackle their snacking habits. Dominic would be a perpetual

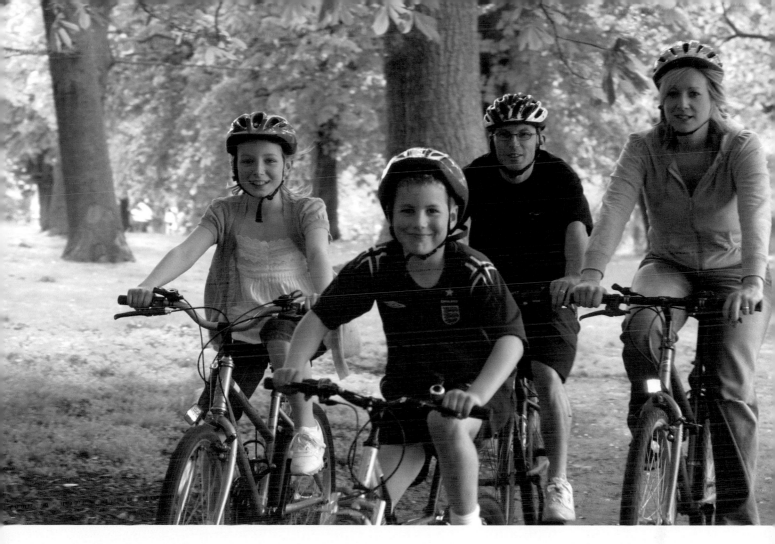

snacker if he could. I've found portion control to be the answer. Instead of buying a big packet of Jaffa cakes I buy those little snack-size 'pods' of mini Jaffas, which Dominic can choose as one of his two daily treats.

Making treats monotonous is another trick. I don't buy five or six sorts of chocolate biscuits anymore – now the children say: 'I'm sick of Penguins, I don't want one.' It really works.

Although we weren't a million miles away from a healthy-weight home, there were still a lot of changes we had to make, like switching to brown rice and wholemeal pasta. When my mum came to stay she said: 'I hate brown rice.' By the time she left she took a packet with her. You need to buy the right type. The brand is the key: some taste better than others. We

WE'VE FOUND THAT LIMITING SCREEN TIME IS ONE OF THE TOUGHEST CHALLENGES OF ALL

also made the switch to wholemeal bread. Before, I'd been buying the white sort with all the goodness left in, but I thought the kids don't know it's not ordinary white bread, so I switched to wholemeal.

Although Mark is super fit and has always eaten whatever he likes – especially outside the home – he knows that he couldn't rely on activity alone to keep healthy. He admitted to me: 'It's easy for me to eat anything I want from a weight point of view – though not from a health one. If I gave up the exercise I do, I'd absolutely balloon if you didn't keep me on the straight and narrow.' He's very honest and says the healthy-weight home is not an idea he would have embraced with open arms. But we can both see the positive difference it's made to our family.

changing your family's lifestyle

There's a surprising amount of science involved in changing your behaviour – it isn't simply a matter of gritting your teeth and getting on with it. Once you know the sound scientific reasons for approaching change in a particular way, you're half way there. This chapter shows you the most successful steps to take towards creating a healthy-weight home. Many people think that weight loss is a behaviour change: in fact, it's the result of changing many different behaviours, including eating and activity.

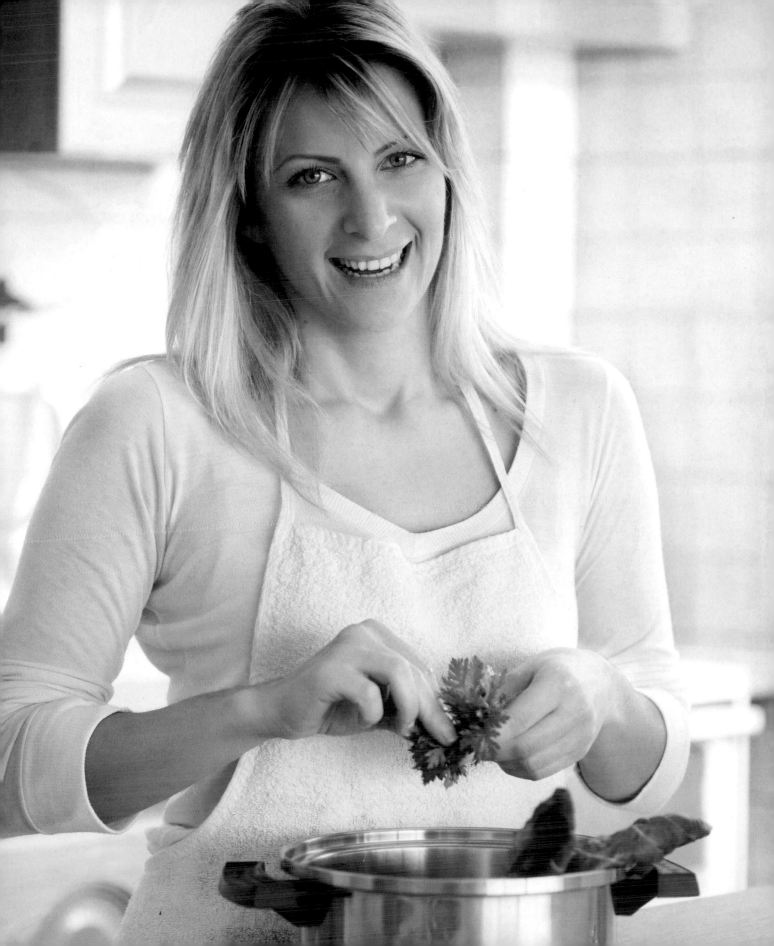

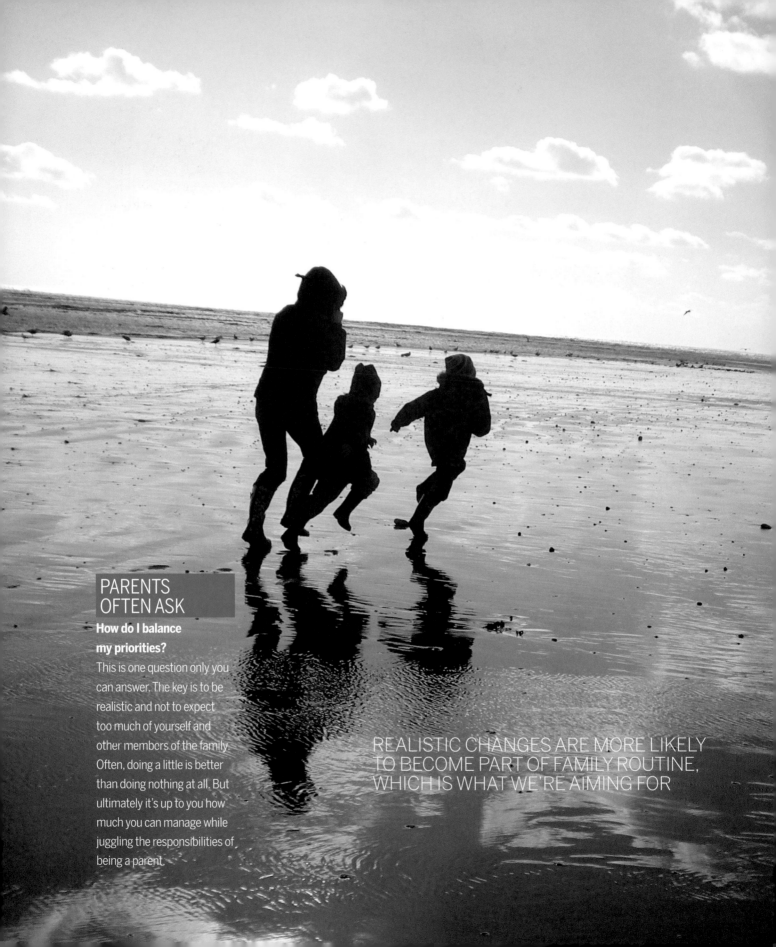

PARENTS OFTEN ASK

How do I balance my priorities?

This is one question only you can answer. The key is to be realistic and not to expect too much of yourself and other members of the family. Often, doing a little is better than doing nothing at all. But ultimately it's up to you how much you can manage while juggling the responsibilities of being a parent.

REALISTIC CHANGES ARE MORE LIKELY TO BECOME PART OF FAMILY ROUTINE, WHICH IS WHAT WE'RE AIMING FOR

The relationship between weight and behaviour

Body weight is affected by everything we do – from how many soft drinks we have to how many hours we spend watching television. If you are gaining weight, the only way to stop is to change some – but not necessarily all – of the behaviours behind the weight gain. Where weight loss is your goal, you need to change more behaviours or make more significant changes to a few key behaviours.

With our already busy lifestyles, just the thought of having to make a big change can often be overwhelming. In the following chapter we are going to give you 5 Simple Rules to help you tackle different areas of your family's life on the way to creating a healthy-weight home. But first we're going to focus on how to make changes in a way that works for everybody in the family.

One step at a time

It's nearly impossible – and it's certainly not recommended – to try to make lots of changes at once. You're much more likely to be successful if you tackle things one at a time. Focusing on changes that are realistic for your family is the best way to start. For example, taking the dog out for a walk before dinner might be something that you could imagine doing comfortably as a family – but you might not be ready to give up going to McDonalds on Fridays. Realistic changes are much more likely to become part of family routine, which is what you're aiming for.

It's also not necessary for you to follow completely all five rules that we're going to give you. Because body weight is determined by literally hundreds, even thousands, of small behaviours, we can pick and choose which strategies to use and how closely to follow them. Consistency in making a few changes is far more likely to lead to lasting success than trying to tackle everything at once.

Be prepared for resistance

Behaviour change is an ongoing process. As parents, we can judge the rate of our family's success over time and, whenever it seems appropriate, we can add more changes to push things along and make greater progress. We can also tell if we've gone too far, and recognise that it might be time to relax a few of the changes until the whole family feels comfortable with progress so far. Trying to force change on the family will only be met with resistance.

PARENTS OFTEN ASK

What if we are ready to change but our children are not?

This is one of the times when being the adult in charge has its advantages. As parents, we set family policies and we are in a position to make changes even when we encounter resistance from our children. The trick is to pick changes in behaviour that will meet with least resistance and then make them in a realistic and consistent way. Over time the struggle gets easier, especially when children see the reality isn't as bad as they expected. And when they start to feel the benefits, there'll be even less resistance to future changes.

The science of change

In the USA, two pioneers in the field of changing behaviour, James Prochaska and Carlo DiClemente, identified five stages to help people decide whether they are ready to change. These stages can help a family decide what steps they are ready to take towards creating a healthy-weight home.

STAGE 1
Pre-contemplation

At this stage change is not even on the family's radar. For example, if the whole family has soft drinks with meals, it hasn't even occurred to any of them to switch to water. The goal of the pre-contemplation stage is to simply get the family thinking about their behaviour. At this stage all the family needs to do is become aware of the behaviours that create a healthy-weight home. Then they can start to think about which specific behaviours they want to tackle.

STAGE 2
Contemplation

This is the time to think about the various behaviours that make up a healthy-weight home and decide which ones your family is happy to change – for example, doing more family activities. But at this stage you won't have a specific plan or timeframe in mind.

STAGE 3
Preparation

Now it's time to look at the ways of actually making changes. It means planning to put changes in action with a specific date in mind. For example, let's say you've decided to switch from soft drinks to water at meal times. If you've already got a stock of soft drinks in the house, you may need to delay the change for a week until it's all used up. On your next trip to the supermarket you need to remember to alter the quantities you buy and maybe choose some sparkling bottled water instead. This will set the scene for successfully making the change at meal times.

This is also a good time to get information on new goals. If you've decided to be more active as a family, then you need to find out what's going on. Look in your local newspaper. Noticeboards in the supermarket, village hall or community centre, health centre or even the newsagent's window will have adverts for yoga classes, Pilates sessions, salsa lessons, sponsored walks, neighbourhood litter-picking sessions, etc.

In the overall change process, preparation should be relatively

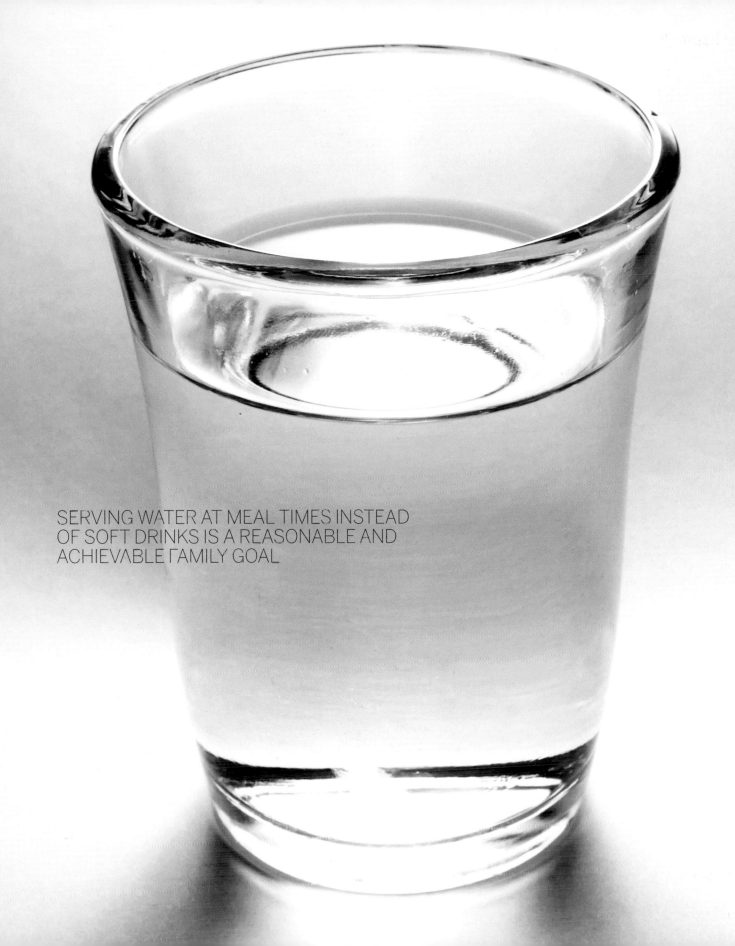

SERVING WATER AT MEAL TIMES INSTEAD
OF SOFT DRINKS IS A REASONABLE AND
ACHIEVABLE FAMILY GOAL

How can I help my children understand the importance of changing their behaviour?

Children with weight issues usually want to lose weight but don't know how to. Explain to them how making small changes to their lifestyle will make a difference to their weight, along with other important benefits like better-fitting clothes and having more energy.

short. You need enough time to work out a realistic plan but, to give yourself the best chance of success, you should aim to start your changes within a month. If start dates repeatedly come and go without being acted on, it's a sign that the change is really still in the contemplation stage and you may well need to go back and rethink your plans.

STAGE 4
Action

Now it's time to put plans into action. A new change may take some time to get used to. Try to stick to the plan for at least several days to help make it happen. Motivation will be high, which increases the chances for success. But it's not uncommon for plans

A FEW IDEAS TO GET YOU STARTED

Increase the number of times you sit down as a family to have dinner together.
Make it something to look forward to. Get some new colourful plates and glasses – Ikea, Matalan, ASDA and Homebase have cheery china that won't break the bank. It's easier to serve new style food on new tableware. Try to make at least one dish a new recipe.

Reduce the number of hours some members of the family spend on the computer.
Start by shifting the computer out of the bedroom, for example – if it's downstairs you can keep an eye on what's going on. Get the children to draw up a timetable so that video or computer games are a treat to be enjoyed after homework or chores. Work

out a daily limit but let family members 'bank' their allowance, so they might have a long session one day but play no games at all another day.

Serve brown rice and wholegrain pasta instead of white rice and pasta.
And increase the amount of salad you eat – salad doesn't have to mean a few limp lettuce leaves and a slice of tomato. Use canned pulses – chick peas, kidney beans, cannellini beans – in salads, along with plenty of chopped flat-leaved parsley, chives or hot leaves like rocket for a satisfying spicy taste.

Serve water with meals instead of soft drinks or fruit juice.
An elegant jug and a new set of glasses can make all the difference, as can ice and lemon.

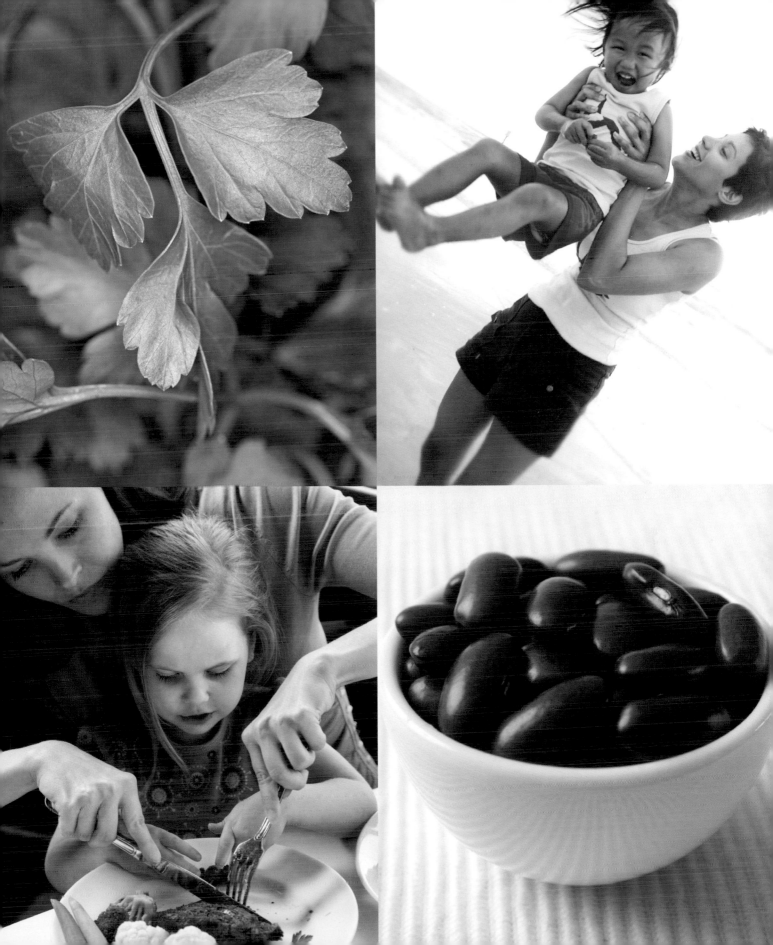

Should everyone in the family have the same goals?

While the main goals should be shared by all family members, there may be different approaches. This is especially true when there are older children in the family – family-based activities don't always appeal to them and they may prefer to join in activities with their friends instead. But being active is still the main goal.

to need modifying. That's ok – it's much easier to tinker with a good plan to make it fit into family life than trying to stick with one that's clearly not working.

STAGE 5
The maintenance phase

Now the change is part of everyday family life. It's simply the way you do things and to make it different would mean making another change. However, you may need to make adjustments every now and then – for example, if you usually go for a walk after dinner, and one of the children joins an evening activity club, then you'll need to rearrange things to take this into account.

Are you ready to change?

Before trying to create a healthy-weight home, you need to get an idea of how ready your family is to make the change. Reluctance to change is not as important as the reasons behind it. For example, your daughter may say she is not ready to have only a couple of treats a day. If you ask why, it may turn out that she is worried about feeling hungry. By understanding that fear, you can see that it might be a good idea to put that change on the back burner for a while and focus on something else, such

as serving up more wholesome nutritious foods – wholewheat pasta dishes, hearty vegetable soups, tuna and borlotti bean salad or lamb casserole with haricot beans (you'll find lots of recipes in Part Four). Because these are so filling, your daughter may get less hungry between meals and so be ready to manage with fewer treats.

Confidence plays a big part in getting ready to change. If you don't have confidence in your own ability to achieve your goal, it can hold you back from trying. As a parent you have to learn to read between the lines. For example, a teenage boy who says he isn't ready to be more active may lack confidence in his ability to cope with some sports. By sitting down and discussing the sort of activities he might enjoy and that are not so physically demanding, as well as being encouraging and supportive, you can boost his confidence.

What do you want to happen?

When planning a change in eating or activity, the first question to ask yourself is: what would I like to happen? Goals can be small and simple, as long as they are realistic and measurable.

Then ask: what needs to happen for the goal to be met? For example, if the goal is to have more family dinners together, the

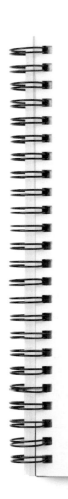

CHECKLIST FOR CHANGE

Get the family together and use this list to help you decide what's right for all of you:

➜ How badly do you want to change?
➜ Will change make a difference to everyday life?
➜ What are the benefits?
➜ Why should you change?
➜ Will it be worth the time and effort?
➜ How will it affect the family's daily routine?
➜ What will the costs be, in money, time and effort?
➜ Are there any advantages to not changing?
➜ What will it feel like to make the change?
➜ What would need to happen to make changing an even higher priority?

GOALS FOR CHANGE

For a successful behaviour change you need four key elements:

➜ A specific realistic goal that can be measured
➜ A plan to achieve the goal
➜ The belief that the goal is important
➜ Confidence that the plan can be carried out

PARENTS OFTEN ASK

What if I'm ready to change but my partner isn't?

This is a tricky one. Forcing anyone – adult or child – to change rarely works. And in many ways it's harder for an adult to change as they've had longer to get used to their own way of doing things. Try to understand why your partner is resistant. If, for example, your partner feels they don't need to change their behaviour, try to help them at least see the benefits your children will gain from creating a healthy-weight home. If they lack confidence, which many adults do, promise them lots of support and encouragement.

plan might include shopping and cooking over the weekend to save time in the week; then letting all family members know that they are expected to be at home for dinner on the days you've chosen; and finally, involving everyone – for example in setting the table and serving the meal.

Deciding how important a goal is and whether it is realistic may need a family discussion. When a family is working towards a common goal everyone has agreed on, the goal is much easier to achieve. To make it a reality, each family member can take responsibility for part of the plan. Parents can cook and freeze the dinners at the weekend; a younger child can set the table, and a teenager can put dinner in the oven when they get in from school.

Finally, the whole family needs to take one last look at the goal and the plan to achieve it. When all the steps are in place it usually becomes clear whether or not a goal is likely to happen.

how to get started

You've decided your family is ready for change – so what's next? Here we present the 5 Simple Rules to help you target different areas of your life. Although the rules are simple we are not suggesting you tackle them all at once. Make changes one at a time, starting with the rule that seems most realistic for your family.

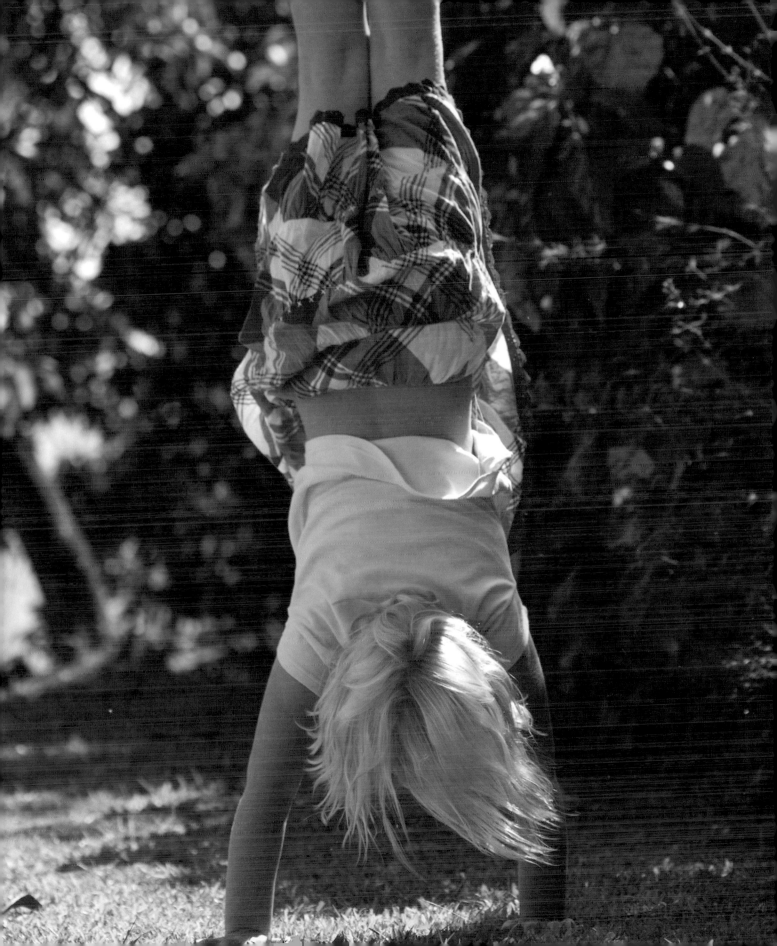

What are the 5 Simple Rules?

RULE 1 Focus on wholesome nutritious foods

RULE 2 Include treats

RULE 3 Limit screen time to a maximum of two hours a day

RULE 4 Try to be active for an hour or more every day

RULE 5 The rules apply to everyone in the home

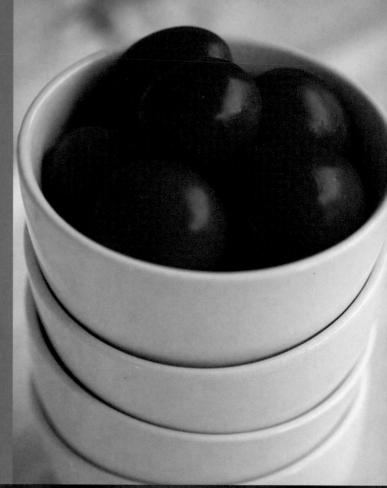

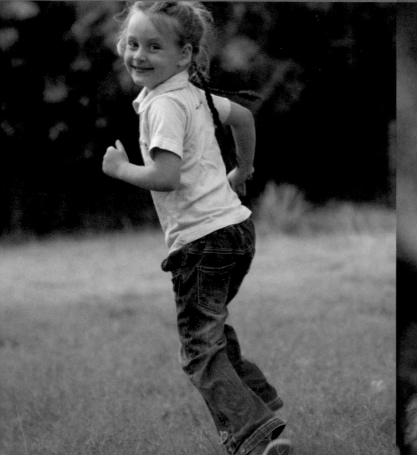

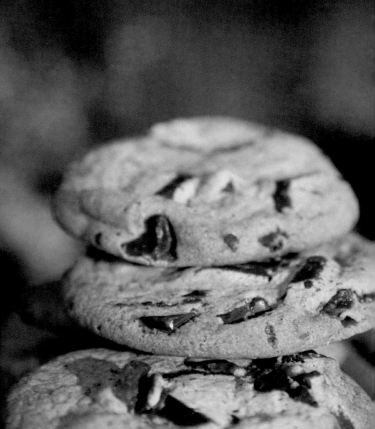

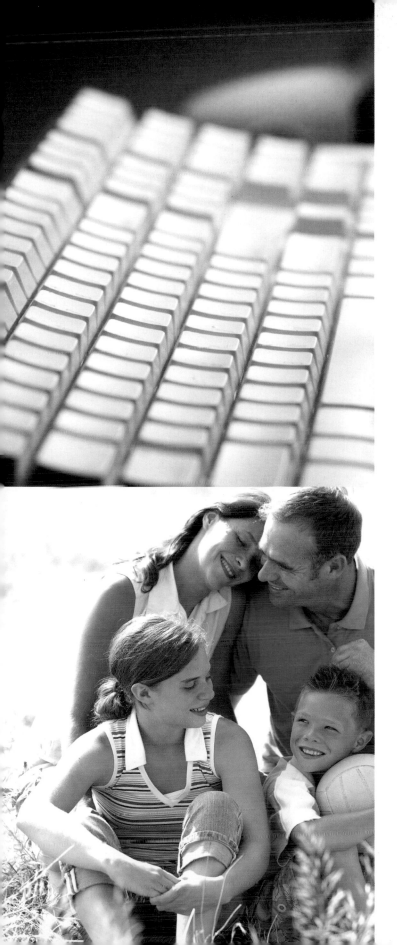

RULE 1 Focus on wholesome nutritious foods

A healthy diet is based on wholesome nutritious foods that are high in vitamins, minerals and other important nutrients, and lower in calories. These foods should be the mainstay of the family's diet and feature in every meal and snack. Basing a diet on these foods not only makes it easier to achieve a healthy weight, it promotes overall health and well-being.

Fruit and vegetables

Fruit and vegetables are packed with all sorts of nutrients. They also contain water and fibre, which help fill you up without supplying too many calories. Filling up on vegetables is a great way to help children eat fewer calories. Government guidelines recommend that everyone eats at least five portions of fruit and vegetables a day. That's at least five – the more you eat, the better. As a rough guide, a portion of fruit is one medium-size apple or banana, a handful of grapes or half a grapefruit. Measure vegetables in tablespoons: one portion is three heaped tablespoons, whether the vegetables are raw, cooked or canned.

Visit the Food Standards Agency

Which of the 5 Simple Rules should I focus on first?

There is no right answer – the best thing to do is to start making the changes that you and your family are ready, willing and able to make. For help on deciding where to start, see Chapter 5.

Breakfast ideas

Poached egg on wholemeal toast

Grilled mushrooms on wholemeal toast

Muesli with skimmed milk and a handful of blueberries

Slices of melon

Grapefruit

Scrambled eggs on wholemeal toast

Low fat yoghurt with chopped fruit

Porridge with dried fruit

healthy eating website for more information at www.eatwell.gov.uk

Cooking with healthy oils

Eating less fat is an effective way to reduce calorie intake but it can reduce the intake of vitamin E, an essential nutrient found in some oils. Cooking with small quantities of healthy oils like rapeseed oil or olive oil will help everyone in the family to get the vitamin E they need. Try making salad dressing with olive oil or sautéing meat and vegetables in rapeseed oil.

Watch out for hidden fats and sugars

Many readymade convenience foods contain extra fats and sugars – not to mention salt – that increase calories without improving nutrition. By preparing simple wholesome meals from basic ingredients you can cut out all those added extras. Lean meats, fresh vegetables and wholegrain foods like pasta take very little time to prepare and are delicious. Look for quick and simple cooking methods such as grilling, sautéing, baking, poaching and steaming. (See recipes in Part Four of this book.)

Family meals

Children who eat dinner at home with their family tend to have a more nutritious diet. They learn how to enjoy a variety of foods, try new foods and learn how to eat healthily. Home-cooked family meals are more nutritionally balanced than restaurant meals or takeaways. Although children love eating at fast-food restaurants, the food on offer is likely to be high in fat and carbohydrates and added sugar, while the drinks available are high in sugar.

Now that cooking is officially cool – thanks to role models like

JUST CHANGE ONE THING

always eat breakfast

Breakfast is an ideal way to kickstart the day, with wholegrain bread or cereal, fruit and calcium-enriched low-fat milk. Research has shown that children who eat breakfast tend to have fewer weight problems than those who skip breakfast. Eating breakfast is also linked to maintaining a healthy weight in adulthood, so making it a regular family meal is a healthy habit that will benefit children in later life. If all the family sits down to breakfast, even better – it promotes togetherness.

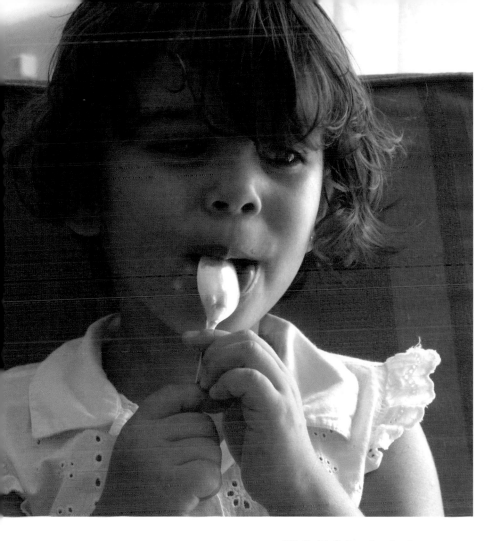

PARENTS OFTEN ASK

I've heard that going on a diet can cause eating disorders. What are the risks if my child follows the 5 Simple Rules?

Healthy Parent, Healthy Child is not a diet book; it's all about following a healthy lifestyle. The 5 Simple Rules and the parenting roles described here can actually help children avoid the emotional triggers that can set off eating disorders. A healthy-weight home is all about eating well and being active without a lot of pressure about body weight, shape or size.

Jamie Oliver and Gordon Ramsay – why not suggest the children make dinner once a week? It needn't actually involve that much 'cooking' – most supermarkets hand out inspirational leaflets and booklets with ideas for putting a few delicious ingredients together to make a quick tasty supper or lunch. The government is also committed to bringing back cookery lessons in secondary schools – and some schools never dropped them from the timetable anyway – so if you have older children you can look forward to tasting their creations.

RULE 2 Include treats

Treats are foods that are high in calories and low in nutrition but taste good. Examples include soft drinks, desserts, chocolate, sweets and highly processed snack foods. But cutting them out all together makes life boring. One or two treats a day adds enjoyment and stops us feeling deprived – treats are part of a realistic eating pattern.

How to include treats in a healthy-weight home

Treats should be part of routine daily life. Don't use them to reward children or to punish them

PARENTS OFTEN ASK

How can children lose weight without actually counting calories?

The extra calories that children eat tend to come from treats. By eating more wholesome nutritious foods and fewer treats, they are automatically reducing the number of calories they eat. And because wholesome foods are more filling too, they are also eating less. If you try to cut calories without looking at what your child is actually eating, they can feel hungry as a result.

JUST CHANGE ONE THING
choose wholegrains

Foods made with wholegrains – like wholewheat or oats – include all parts of the kernel, which contains most of the vitamins and minerals. Wholemeal or wholegrain bread, brown rice, wholewheat pasta and wholegrain cereal are also full of fibre, which helps keep the intestine healthy and – very important – makes you feel full up. A diet rich in fibre is recommended for children and adults and can reduce the chances of constipation – a common childhood problem.

Substitute brown rice for white rice; wholemeal or wholegrain bread for white bread; wholewheat pasta for white pasta; and choose wholegrain breakfast cereals. Do it in small steps at first if you like, mix white and wholewheat pasta together so that everyone gets used to the texture, colour and taste.

– research has shown that this approach makes treats even more desirable to children, making them even more of a minefield to deal with. Instead, aim to show them that treats can be a special but regular part of everyday eating.

Exactly what constitutes a treat varies from person to person, and can be influenced by age, mood and other factors. It's up to each member of the family to decide what their treat food should be. While you might choose a glass of wine with dinner, your six-year-old will prefer a chocolate bar.

Treat or snack?

It's very important to differentiate between treats and snacks. Children need snacks because their stomachs are too small to hold enough food to last from meal to meal. Think of a snack as a mini-meal to keep your child going: it should be wholesome and nutritious, such as a banana or a slice of wholemeal toast.

Portion size

Along with the rise in weight problems has come a corresponding increase in portion size. Food portions in restaurants and fast-food chains can be up to eight times bigger than recommended. Our children have grown up in a world of large portions so that a 500ml bottle of soft drink (that's a pint of lemonade, for example) and a supersize chocolate bar seems

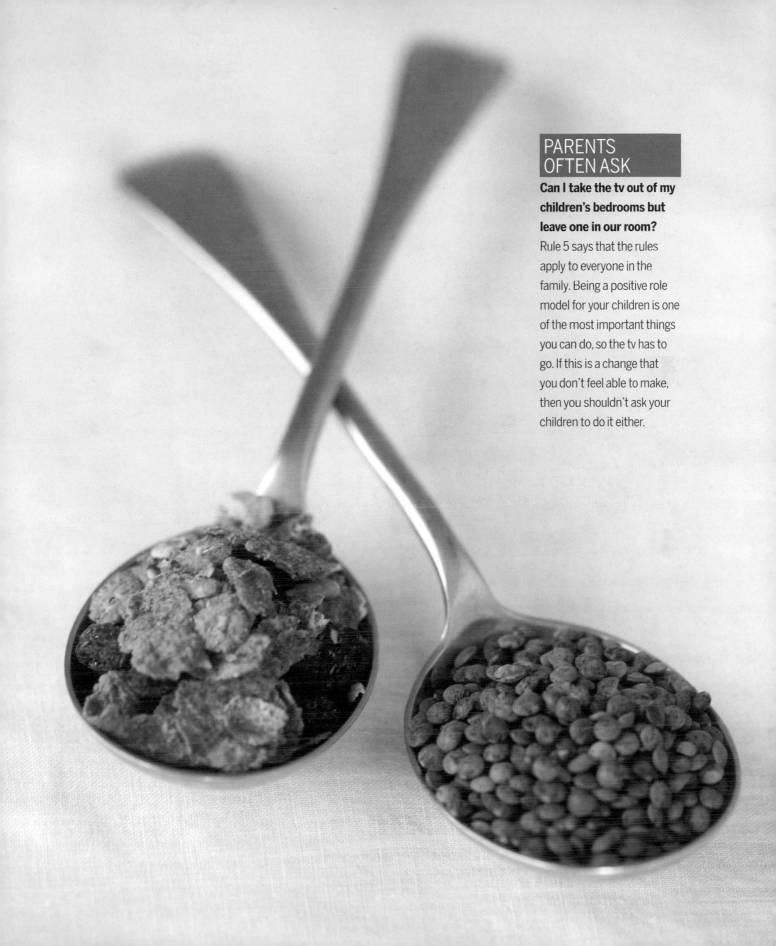

PARENTS OFTEN ASK

Can I take the tv out of my children's bedrooms but leave one in our room?

Rule 5 says that the rules apply to everyone in the family. Being a positive role model for your children is one of the most important things you can do, so the tv has to go. If this is a change that you don't feel able to make, then you shouldn't ask your children to do it either.

If my child plays a sport or has swimming lessons or tennis or dance lessons, isn't that enough activity in their life?

Probably not. Most sports teams and lessons involve only a few hours activity a week, which falls short of the hour a day recommendation in Rule 4. To get a better idea, monitor how much time they spend actually doing the activity – not standing around watching – and see how it adds up.

JUST CHANGE ONE THING

drink water, low-fat milk or low-calorie drinks

Cutting out high-sugar soft drinks can make a huge difference. A UK study showed that children who simply cut back on soft drinks lost weight over the course of a year, while a control group who carried on drinking them actually gained weight. And fruit juice isn't as nutritious as you might think – although it contains nutrients, it's high in calories.

normal to them. Research has confirmed that when children are served large portions – surprise, surprise – they tend to eat more. That's another good reason to eat at home most of the time.

RULE 3 Limit screen time to a maximum of two hours a day

Computers, dvds, video games and television are an inescapable part of modern life. More than a quarter of school-age children watch at least four hours of television a day and sitting in front of the tv has been linked to weight gain. And research has shown that adults who watched more television as children weigh more than and are less fit than adults who watched less television in their early years.

It goes without saying that sitting in front of a screen uses up far fewer calories than going outside and playing.

Keep the tv out of the bedroom

Children who have a tv in their bedroom are even more likely to develop weight problems, probably because watching tv is so convenient and accessible. If possible don't have tvs, computers or video game consoles in a child's bedroom where you can't monitor their use.

If children need to use a computer for homework, their screen time allowance of two hours is on top of homework use.

RULE 4 Try to be active for an hour or more every day

Most children currently get around 30 minutes of activity a day – that's half the recommended level. Experts agree that this is not enough to prevent excess weight gain or to help weight loss. An hour a day may sound like a lot of activity to schedule in, but it isn't when you realise that it includes all sorts of unstructured activity as well as organised sports sessions, etc. Everything from cycling down to the shop to playing outside after school counts towards the total.

Don't leave it to schools
Schools don't always have the resources to make sure children get the activity they need. As children grow up, the time they spend actively playing tends to go down – this is especially true of any children with weight issues. Science shows that the home is the most influential factor in changing children's habits.

Listen to your children
Activity can be a good opportunity for some family fun. Ask your children what they'd like to do. Don't just sign them up for a sport. Asking them to choose may improve the commitment and motivation they have. Many children prefer unstructured play:

research shows that walking, for example, is a great way to get them off the sofa and out of the house.

RULE 5 **The rules apply to everyone in the home**
A healthy-weight lifestyle is not just for the children or those family members who have weight issues. The rules work if everyone in the family follows them. All family members – whether they are at a healthy weight or not – will benefit from the healthy lifestyle that the rules promote.

Anyone who cares for children needs to get involved too. Childminders, grandparents, preschool groups – all have a big influence. Tell them about the 5 Simple Rules and give them clear information on everything they need to know, from giving children healthy snacks and meals, to limiting screen time and being more active.

PARENTS OFTEN ASK
Shouldn't children drink full-fat milk? And surely 100% fruit juice is good for them?
Children over the age of two don't need the calories or saturated fats in full-fat milk. They should have low-fat calcium-enriched dairy products. And while the vitamins and minerals in fruit juice are good for them, fruit juice contains a lot of calories without filling them up. It's better for kids to get the same vitamins and minerals from a piece of fresh fruit.

JUST CHANGE ONE THING
regular meals and snacks
Eating meals at regular times has been shown to improve healthy eating. Children from families that don't sit down to regular meals tend to snack more frequently on high-calorie treats. Be ready when the children come bursting in after school – have a bowl of fruit on the table or carrot sticks and celery in the fridge with a low-fat dip. Or have snack packs of dried fruit and nuts handy in the cupboard and hide the biscuit tin away.

case study 3

Debbie Court and her husband Darren have five children: Louis age 7, Georgia 10, Lana 11, Ryan 13 and Ross 15. Creating a healthy-weight home has taken some effort but now the 5 Simple Rules have become part of family life and no one really stops to think about them any more

Darren and I have always been health conscious and so some of the steps to creating a healthy-weight home came naturally. As we were already eating nutritious food, that seemed the easiest place to start – by tweaking our menu a bit further to make it even healthier. The first thing I did was to switch to wholegrains instead of carrying on serving white bread and pittas and white pasta. Wherever possible I made the change easier by serving half and half – a 50:50 mix of wholemeal and white pasta, for example. I used the same trick for switching from Frosties to cornflakes – though it didn't work for everyone in the family. Children can be acute at detecting change.

The next thing I did was to introduce more choice at meal times and to let everyone serve themselves. I really had to stop myself plating up their meals. Because I knew what each child would and wouldn't eat, I'd got used to 'customising' their dinner plates: I wouldn't put something on if I thought they wouldn't eat it. Ryan was a case in point: he would only eat peas, and I had to disguise onions in a dish by chopping them so finely they were practically invisible. I remember when he first served himself one green bean. I nearly fell off my chair. After he ate it, he said: 'You know mum, that was all right.'

As with many families, reducing screen time was the biggest challenge. For example, Louis found it hard to realise that screen time didn't just mean watching tv. I had to make him understand he couldn't just switch off the telly and switch on his Nintendo.

It was really hard in the winter. When it's raining, grim and dark, the first thing you want to do is come in and switch on the tv. Once the children are in front of it they go brain dead; you speak to them and they don't even answer. To distract them, Darren and I got games out, things we'd almost forgotten, like Monopoly, draughts, chess and Twister. For the younger ones, colouring books and crafts activities were great for tempting them away from the telly.

Although we had a basketball post, we used to keep it tucked away so that it wouldn't get stolen, so if any one wanted to play with it, they had to drag it onto the middle of the drive. Just making the decision to keep it on the drive and instantly accessible has made it so much easier for the boys to go out and shoot a few balls. A small change that's made a big difference.

Family cookery sessions are a great way to distract the children and there are all sorts of benefits, such as helping them make healthy food choices and boosting their confidence by letting them get tea ready. I let all five of them loose on making fruit salad, now I've stopped worrying about the sharp knives. It's a great

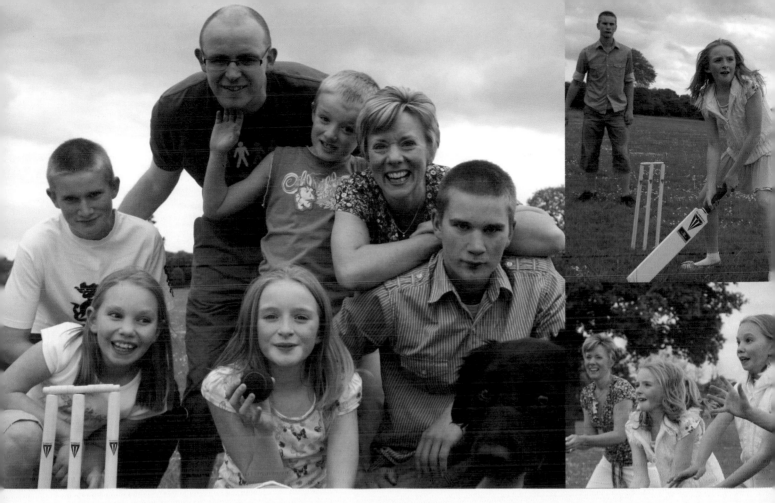

way to encourage children to try different fruits. Before we started, most of the children wouldn't eat anything other than apples, and even those had to be chopped, with the core cut out.

Louis is setting a bit of a trend at school with his packed lunches – his friends like to look in his lunchbox and see what he's got. Mums have come up to me and told me that their children have started asking why they can't take pitta bread and dips to school like Louis? Even the dinner ladies like to take a peek and see what he's eating.

Before we started following the 5 Simple Rules, both Ryan and I had had weight problems. I had just lost 5st 5lb with Weight Watchers and Ryan had lost 1st 11lb. The idea of the healthy-weight home came along at just the right time for us. Unusually for a teenager, Ryan had lost weight by going to WeightWatchers

ONCE YOU'VE LOST WEIGHT, YOU'LL KEEP IT OFF EFFORTLESSLY LIVING IN A HEALTHY-WEIGHT HOME

meetings (with our GP's approval), but he hadn't exactly enjoyed following a diet.

Now he's got the weight off, he can keep it off effortlessly by living in a healthy-weight home. It's also made a massive difference to Ryan's asthma – he hasn't used an inhaler since we started.

Going for a walk with the dog is my 'me' time. When I lost weight I bought her especially for me. She's a labrador/collie cross so I knew she'd need lots of walking. We walk for miles and have got much faster.

I love going out as a family too – we like going bowling or on a family bike ride. We didn't use to do things together before, I'm not sure why – I just don't think we realised that we could.

When I see the difference a healthy-weight home has made to my family, I think 'Wow.' I'm 110 per cent behind it and I want to tell everyone about the benefits.

part 2

positive
action

the roles parents play

There are all sorts of ways we can encourage our children to eat healthily, whatever their age, from being a good food role model and leading by example, to stocking the kitchen with healthy food, setting meal times and getting everyone – from babes in arms to rebellious teenagers – eating together. The roles you need to adopt as a parent are:

1 The Food Role Model

2 The Food Provider

3 The Food Enforcer

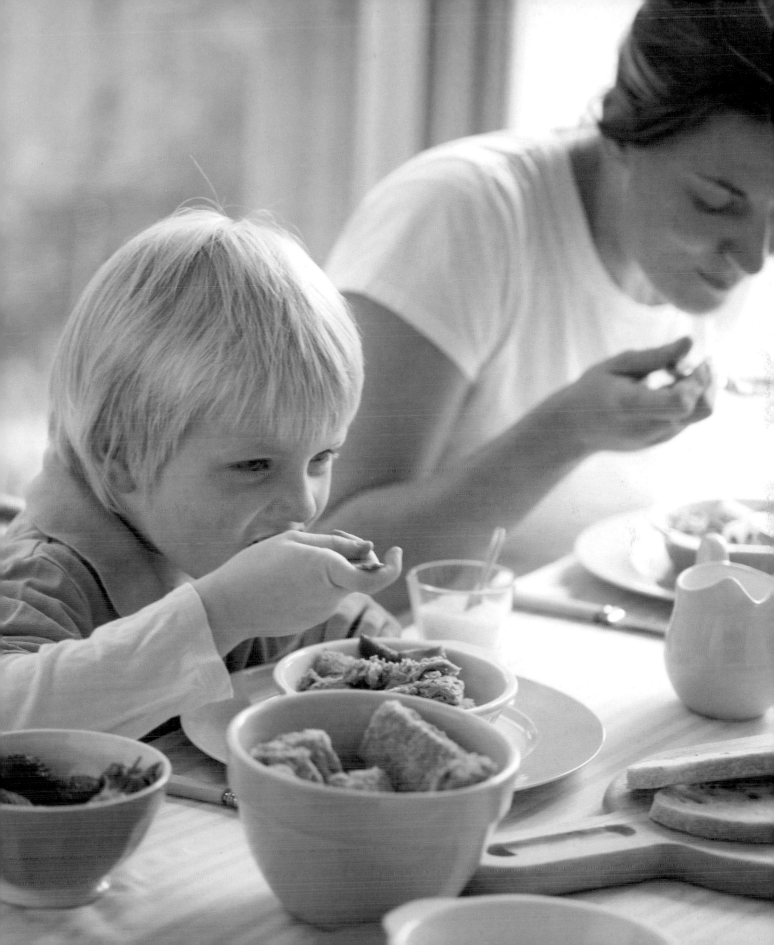

Remember the 5 Simple Rules

Rule 1: Focus on wholesome nutritious foods

Rule 2: Include treats

Rule 3: Limit screen time to a maximum of two hours a day

Rule 4: Try to be active for an hour or more every day

Rule 5: The rules apply to everyone in the home

In this chapter you'll find lots of ways of putting Rules 1 and 2 into practice. These vary according to a child's age – you need to come up with different ideas for babies, toddlers, young children and older children.

The food role model

➔ Eats wholesome nutritious foods

➔ Enjoys treats in moderation

➔ Understands the importance of family meals

➔ Shows that healthy eating is part of feeling good about yourself and taking care of yourself

As parents we have a huge effect on our children's eating habits, influencing what they like to eat, how much they eat and even when they eat. We also pass on our attitudes to food: if you eat a proper breakfast every day, it's likely your children will too.

Being a good role model for food and eating habits means following the 5 Simple Rules consistently and with a positive attitude. To create a healthy-weight home we have to take on the responsibility for family eating, working side by side with our partners and children to practise healthy eating without blaming or punishing each other. And healthy eating doesn't have to mean dull or worthy food – you may be surprised at how tasty and varied your menus will become if you follow the rules and try some of the recipes in Part Four of this book.

Being a good role model gives us the chance to show by example that working towards a healthy-weight home fits easily into everyday life. If we follow the 5 Simple Rules it shows our children that we have a positive opinion of ourselves – and this will encourage their own feelings of self worth. Lots of different behaviour falls under the category of food role model and our actions are constantly on show, from which snacks we choose, to which treats we like, to how we present a meal.

> **JUST CHANGE ONE THING**
>
> Put treats in a container on a high shelf, not at eye level. There's a lot to be said for 'out of sight, out of mind.'

> **JUST CHANGE ONE THING**
>
> Small, gradual changes work best. Here are some ideas. Tried and tested steps to begin with include switching from oil to a cooking-oil spray for sautéing; having reduced-fat milk and water at meal times instead of soft drinks; buying extra-lean mince; choosing wholewheat pasta instead of white and brown rice instead of white; and buying more fresh fruit and vegetables.

The food provider

→ Establishes regular meal and snack times
→ Buys and prepares food
→ Decides where meals are eaten
→ Has a positive attitude to food
→ Is consistent about food
→ Creates a happy atmosphere at the table

What is a food provider? The short answer is you. Food providers are in charge of the family's schedule, deciding what time meals and snacks are served and where they are eaten. They decide which foods to buy and how much food to keep in the cupboards and fridge/freezer at home.

Limiting treats

Limiting the number and types of treats in the house is an effective way of dealing with them. It's hard to argue with a child about whether a treat is permitted or not, if you haven't actually got any. Not having too many treats in the cupboard helps us adults to be better food role models.

All of us, children and adults, will find something we want to eat if we are really hungry. Most children tend to be a bit lazy and will eat whatever food is quick, easy and available. So if they find biscuits, they will eat biscuits. If they find yoghurts, fresh fruit – the ultimate convenience food – and carrot sticks, then that's what they'll eat. A strategy that works for many families is to keep the wholesome foods at the front of the fridge or at eye level in the cupboard and store treats in hard-to-reach places.

While limiting the range of treats works, banning treats outright doesn't. A middle-of-the-road approach with a few treats available is best. While it may make economic sense, treats really shouldn't be bought in bulk – this makes sticking to Rule 2 easier.

Many of us think that if we simply don't let our children have any treats they will learn not to want them. Unfortunately this strategy usually backfires. Research shows that banning or putting extreme limits on treats tends to have the opposite effect: children will want

Research shows that banning or putting extreme limits on treats tends to have the opposite effect: children will want them more, not less.

Shopping for treats

Rob does the family's weekly shop and he was worried what the children would say when he came home with fewer treats than usual.

Parents can worry unnecessarily about how their children are going to react. Often the reality is much easier to deal with than the imagined scenario. Most children will eat healthy snacks without much fuss – especially if that's all that is available. They adjust quickly to having a limited number of treats and soon grasp the concept of when they're gone, they're gone.

Healthy snacks can be made more appealing by offering children a choice: for example, a bowl of popcorn or a bowl of cereal. By giving a set choice rather than asking 'What would you like for a snack?' you're setting the stage for one or the other to be selected. Rob was delighted to find this tactic works and his initial fears were groundless.

How to recognise hunger

Sylvia knew it was a good idea if her 10-year-old daughter Alice had something to eat rather than getting too hungry. On the other hand she didn't want to ruin her appetite by giving her too many snacks between meals.

One of the best things you can do for your children is help them to recognise true feelings of hunger. Even quite small children can be helped to work this out but older children can discuss it readily. Sylvia asked Alice if she really was hungry or whether she just felt like eating. If it was the latter, they talked about what had made her want to eat and found things to do to take her mind off it until the next meal. She got Alice to rate her hunger and if it was intense she gave her a snack. If she rated her hunger as medium and dinner was nearly ready, she encouraged her to wait. As time went on Alice learned to judge her feelings of hunger and could work out for herself if she needed a snack or could wait until dinner.

them more, not less. If the ban is strictly enforced, children are also likely to sneak treats into the house – and the last thing we want to do is create a closet chocoholic.

It's easier to be a food provider when you're cooking meals at home. It's more difficult when you're eating out: although you can suggest a restaurant that has healthy options on the menu, obviously you have far less control over what's eaten. In order to stick to Rule 1, many families find it easier to cook simple meals at home and eat out less frequently.

Getting the balance right

Let your children decide how much they want to eat, to match their feelings of fullness and hunger. Doing this helps children to learn to eat only when they are truly hungry and to stop when they are full. You can ask your children questions to help them decide and to teach them to learn to recognise when they feel hungry. Asking a child who's just got in from school: 'Are you hungry? Would you like a snack?' will help them decide whether they are hungry or not, rather than assuming they need a snack out of habit.

As food providers we need to find the right balance between setting regular meal and snack times and being flexible enough to respond

JUST CHANGE ONE THING

Sit down to dinner as often as you can. The family meal is one of the most important strategies you can insist on as an enforcer to create a healthy-weight home. Research shows that children who eat family dinners are likely to eat more vegetables, fruit and dairy products than children who don't. They are also more likely to eat breakfast.

to real feelings of hunger. The policies we set up affect everyone in the home. For example, you may decide that food can only be eaten in the kitchen and dining room; that the tv is turned off when dinner is served; and salad will be on the menu every day. Being consistent gives children the structure they want and need. Gradually, over time, these policies will become part of the way your family functions and part of the daily routine. And any exceptions will seem strange – even unwanted – to family members.

As part of our role as food provider we have the chance to get our families to try new foods, such as asparagus, artichokes and mangoes. And we can take them to new restaurants such as a sushi bar or a Thai restaurant. Expanding your healthy food options is a great strategy because it helps the whole family to enjoy eating without ignoring the basics of a healthy-weight home.

The food enforcer

→ Sets the rules and their order of priority

→ Is consistent but not rigid

→ Creates the family food environment

→ Promotes healthy food choices

→ Is a positive influence

→ Supports the family's food and eating behaviours

→ Counteracts negative influences

What is a food enforcer? Again the answer is you, whether you realise it or not. As a parent you set the house rules – everything from insisting everyone makes their bed each morning to deciding what you drink with dinner. Parents are the enforcers. Being an effective enforcer can be challenging: there's a fine line between imposing the rules too strictly and not being tough enough when they are broken.

Children need structure and nowhere is this more essential than in family life. Structure provides the framework children need to build their lives – and it needs a strong foundation. It's a bit like a house: think of the walls and foundations

as the structure, which the children then decorate with their own personality and style.

But children also need flexibility. How much depends on how old they are, and increases as they grow from babies to young adults. The process of growing up doesn't go smoothly. Children fight against house rules as a way of gaining more freedom and room to change. Just as it's our job to enforce the rules, it's the child's job to protest against them.

Setting food policies

In a healthy-weight home the food enforcer makes sure everyone sticks to the family eating policies. We parents decide how the 5 Simple Rules will work in our family. We create the boundaries and enforce them consistently. We decide what time meals and snacks are served, and which foods are treats. The goal of being an enforcer is not to join the food police, but to make sure that the family is behaving in a way that promotes good health, well-being and a healthy weight. The role of food enforcer focuses on those foods and eating behaviours that affect the whole family.

Be consistent

Many parents find the rules that focus on positive action, like eating

Cutting down on treats

Peter and Jan joined a weight-loss programme and in an effort to cut down on their calorie intake, they bought low-fat or low-sugar versions of their favourite treats. Soon the whole family was tucking into low-fat ice cream and reduced-fat crisps but the thought did occur to them that this might not be the right approach to a healthy-weight home.

Switching to low-fat, low-sugar versions of your favourite foods is a good start but the fact is that they are still treats and ultimately the whole family benefits from shifting the focus from treats to more wholesome foods. If there are too many treats in the house, most people will eat them too often. By buying more fruit and healthy snacks such as wholegrain biscuits and cereal bars, Peter and Jan managed to get the family to enjoy more nutritious foods.

Equal treatment

Judith was trying to create a healthy-weight home for her children but she decided not to include her husband Phil as he worked late shifts and usually brought home a take-away for his dinner. But one day he came home early and the children wanted to know why daddy was having Chinese and they weren't.

It's Rule 5 again – the rules apply to everyone in the home. By sticking to Rule 5, no one feels resentful or left out and everyone in the family benefits.

more wholesome nutritious foods or getting more exercise, easy to enforce. It can be harder to find effective ways to enforce rules that limit treats or screen time – this is where being an enforcer can be challenging.

Consistency is a key aspect. If it means not following all of the 5 Simple Rules to perfection, then so be it. It's better to be consistent in the aspects that are most important to your family. When it comes to creating a healthy-weight home, doing a little all of the time will get you further towards your goal than doing a lot inconsistently.

Young children look to us as the source of food. They have a natural trust that they will be given the right foods in the right amounts and at the right time of day. This trust shapes a child's attitude to food. Children are very self-centred and don't realise that their parents and childminders have busy lives and need to make daily compromises. Many mums have a hard time balancing family life with work, while trying to create a happy home and make sure everyone eats healthily. Consistently providing wholesome nutritious food to eat despite all the odds sends a powerful message to children at any early age.

As children get older, consistency continues to be very important.

The types and amounts of foods in the house affect every family member's diet. In one study it was found that girls ate more fruit and vegetables simply because they were available at home. The same study showed that easy access to less wholesome foods meant that family members made less healthy choices: for example, girls who could help themselves to soft drinks at home ate far fewer dairy products.

Be positive

An enforcer can turn potentially negative situations into positive ones. One way is to focus on telling children what they can do, rather than telling them what they can't do. For example, instead of saying 'You can't have any fruit juice to drink,' try rephrasing: 'Since you're thirsty, I'll get you some water.'

> When it comes to creating a healthy-weight home, doing a little all of the time will get you further towards your goal than doing a lot inconsistently.

When offering snacks, get your child to choose between, say, a peanut butter sandwich or an apple with some cheese. This type of positive enforcing takes a lot of practice but it's well worth it.

Limiting treats

It can be hard to enforce rules about limiting treats. Here are two effective strategies. Buy treat foods in single servings and allow children to choose their treat for the day. One mum turned choosing treats into an afternoon activity by walking to the shop with her children and letting them choose something for themselves. She found this approach stopped the children from becoming obsessed with sweets at home.

If children are allowed to choose treats they are much more careful about their own decisions, such as whether to have a biscuit after school or before bedtime. Avoid putting pressure on your children by telling them not to eat certain treats when they are at friends' houses. The end result is that the children usually end up eating more of the foods than if they'd never been mentioned.

Don't overdo it

It's easy to overdo the role of food enforcer with the best intentions. But superstrict rules rarely work. Research has shown that girls' eating habits in particular can be adversely affected by parents – especially mothers – who are too strict about food. The enforcer should be aiming for a healthy balance between foods.

In a healthy-weight home everyone needs to follow the same rules. While the 5 Simple Rules are simple, they are not easy. As parents we often have trouble enforcing our own eating habits: we try to be too strict, too rigid, too perfect – then end up overeating.

Many of us don't realise just how much our own eating patterns affect our children's habits and ultimately their weight. One study showed that preschool children whose mothers went through periods of overeating struggled with self control themselves. In another study children whose parents were at either end of the scale – either extremely strict about what they ate or had periods of uncontrolled eating – had more body fat than children whose parents did neither. Preschool children whose parents' behaviour went from one extreme to the other gained most body fat of all.

How do we have such an effect on our children?

It's partly to do with being a role model, when we lead by example. Without realising it, it's easy for us to apply some of our own restrictive eating patterns to our children. To reduce the chances of this happening it really helps if we stop and think about what we eat. If you yourself are overweight you might find it helpful to join a weight-loss programme like Weight Watchers, where you'll learn healthy eating habits and positive thinking, and benefit from the supportive atmosphere.

putting the roles into action

Being a parent means taking on many roles as the previous chapter demonstrated, but how do we put them into action? As children develop from babies to toddlers to teens, we need different strategies to cope with each stage. Here's how to put theory into practice.

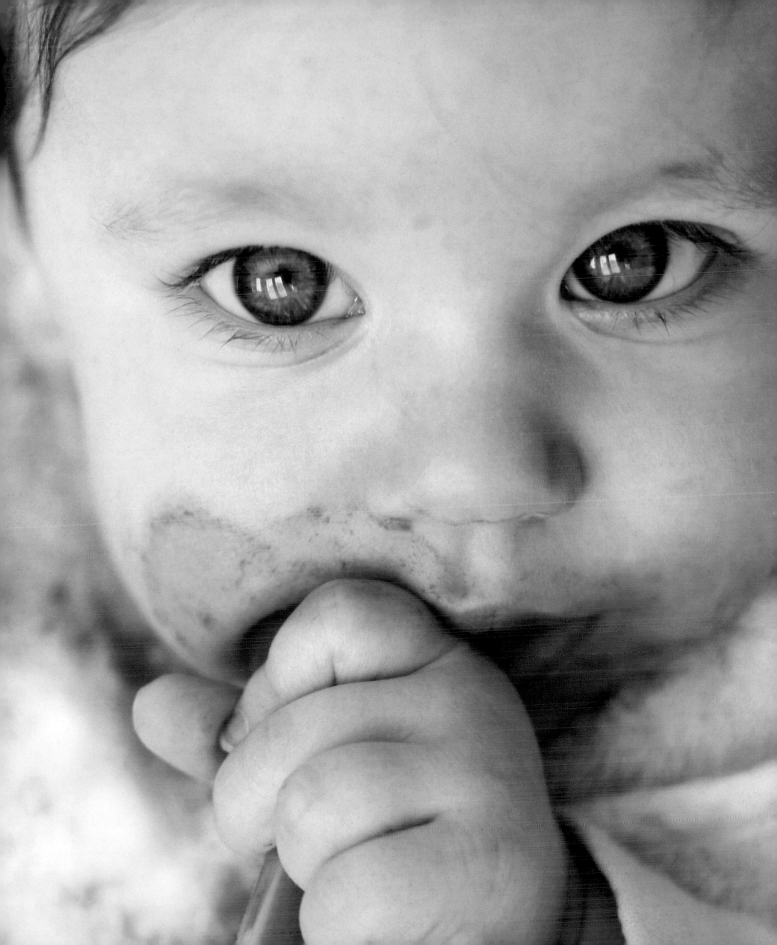

Starting solids

Sarah was worried that her 10-month-old son Jack showed no interest in solid foods and preferred his bottle.

It turned out that baby Jack hadn't had much opportunity to watch other people eating. The family routine was to feed him before mealtimes and then leave him to have a nap or play while they sat at the table. But it's never too early to include babies in meal times. So for the next week Jack joined the family for meals and he had his bottle while everyone else ate. As the days went by he watched everyone else eating and enjoying their food and began to lose interest in his bottle, while becoming very interested in what everyone else had on their plates. Within weeks Jack was happily eating the same foods as his brother and sister. All members of the family, even his siblings, were acting as food role models for baby Jack.

babies

Being a food role model for babies

It's easy to underestimate how much babies absorb and how quickly they learn to copy what we do. It's never too early to start a healthy eating routine.

Looking and learning

As soon as they can, babies keep a close eye on what's going on around them. They watch what their parents, carers and other children are doing. Although babies are limited to breast milk or formula milk for around the first six months, they are already learning eating habits before they even take their first bite. So it makes sense to include babies in family meal times as soon as possible.

Babies get their first lessons in how to eat by watching others. In fact, a sign that a baby is ready to start solids is a growing interest in what everyone else is eating – some babies will even grab at the food. Most babies are ready to start solids at around six months old.

Meals that include a variety of foods teach children about the concept of a balanced diet and the importance of eating foods from all the food groups. Babies can learn what a meal looks like – different colours and shapes – even though they may be too young to try all the foods on the plate.

Sending out messages

Once babies start to eat the same food as everyone else, they quickly catch on if they think they are being manipulated to get them to eat something. Making a big deal about food with words or body language affects a child's attitude to that food – both positively and negatively. Saying, 'This broccoli is very good for you' when you want

JUST CHANGE ONE THING

Don't force your baby to eat. Research shows that babies who are encouraged or coaxed to finish a bottle or a meal – or to eat when they are not hungry – are more likely to gain excess weight. Not only does this habit mean that babies are taking in more calories than their bodies need, it can actually disrupt how they learn to tell when they are full up – by overriding their natural feelings of fullness. This can affect a child's ability to eat the right amounts of food when they are older.

your child to eat it up – or an older brother or sister pulling a face when broccoli is served – sends a message that this food is not to be trusted. It doesn't take long for a baby to work out that the 'Yum' that comes with ice cream and the frown that greets broccoli mean that ice cream is something you want while broccoli is not. For this reason experts recommend that we should react neutrally and equally to all types of food.

Start with Rule 1

As soon as your baby starts on solids, Rule 1 should kick in: focus on wholesome nutritious foods. If possible make your own baby foods at home by puréeing fruit and veg, and freezing individual portions in ice-cube trays. You can purée or mash fruit and veg that you've cooked for the rest of the family as long as you haven't added any salt or sugar. Try making a smooth purée of carrot, parsnip, potato or yam, or a fruit purée such as banana, cooked apple, pear or mango. Babies can also have cereals such as baby rice, sago, maize, cornmeal or millet – but no wheat until they are older.

If you buy readymade baby foods – and we all need to from time to time – make sure that they have been prepared without added fat or sugar. Baby foods with added sugar or fat can lead to your child developing a preference for high-calorie low-nutrient foods.

Make meal times pleasant

Enjoyable family meals are about more than good table manners. They're about sitting down together, having a conversation and focusing on each other without the distraction of tv or radio. If your family is in the habit of eating in front of the tv, set a goal to see if you can manage a week without the tv and eat each meal around the table together. At the end of a week set another goal to see if you can manage two weeks until it becomes second nature.

Even when a baby is too young to sit at the table, the same guidelines apply. Whoever is feeding the baby should concentrate on what they're doing without keeping an eye on the tv or listening to music. The baby can become just as distracted as you and this can mean that both of you may miss the signs that the baby has had enough to eat.

BABIES ARE ALREADY LEARNING EATING HABITS BEFORE THEY EVEN TAKE THEIR FIRST BITE

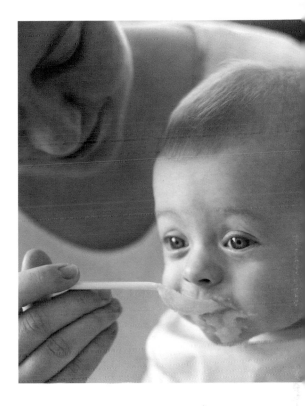

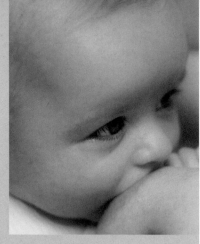

Breastfeeding or bottle?

New mums have to decide whether to breastfeed or bottle feed their baby. There is strong scientific evidence for the advantages of breastfeeding, which include boosting the baby's immune system, helping brain development and reducing the risk of a child becoming overweight. Because the baby is also effectively in control of how much milk they have, they are more likely to match their intake to the calories they need. There is also evidence that breastfed babies who get to taste a variety of foods via their mothers' milk are more receptive to a greater variety of foods when they start on solids. There's a bonus for mums too: breastfeeding can also help them get back to their pre-pregnancy weight more quickly.

While there are benefits to breastfeeding, it is not the right choice for every mother – or every baby. Bottle feeding (using expressed breast milk or formula) is a perfectly acceptable way to feed babies, and bottle-fed babies grow and develop normally.

Being a food provider for babies

Babies know when they want to feed and when they want to stop. We need to learn to recognise and respond to these signs.

Learn to understand your baby

To help babies develop their natural senses of hunger and fullness that they were born with we need to understand their reactions. This applies equally to breastfed and bottle-fed babies. If your baby turns away from the breast, then stop feeding. Similarly, take the bottle away when your baby begins to lose interest, even if the bottle isn't empty.

Once babies are ready to start eating solid food, begin by giving them very small portions and follow your baby's hunger and fullness cues. It can be difficult to feed a baby until you understand their reactions. Babies often frown and make faces when given a new food; they may refuse it or even spit it out. This is a perfectly natural reaction to something new and doesn't mean they will never eat this food. Research has shown that babies need to be given a new food repeatedly before they accept it.

Faddy eating

A leading UK psychologist has done some research into the origins of faddy eating that emphasises the importance of introducing a wide range of foods to babies during weaning. By the time they are toddlers it's almost too late: toddlers already have a range of food they know and recognise but are much more resistant to new foods. This is thought to be an evolutionary benefit: young children and toddlers are reluctant to put foods that they don't recognise in their mouths, to avoid the risk of poisoning.

By introducing a good range of textures and tastes from six months, babies get used to different tastes and textures and learn the motor skills of eating. By the time they are one year old they have their own visual images of safe acceptable foods. And the more foods they find acceptable at this stage, the more foods they are likely to accept as they grow up – this is an influence that can be traced from weaning right up to age seven.

Being a food enforcer for babies

Babies are dependent on us for food so enforcement at this age is automatic – we don't even think about it. But we may not realise how much our own actions can influence a baby's eating habits.

How it works

When a new mum has decided to breastfeed, she needs support from everyone else around her – including her partner and other caregivers. Breastfeeding gives a baby a good start in the healthy-weight home: research shows that breastfed babies drink fewer sweetened drinks and prefer foods with less added sugar as they get older. But you have to have support. For example, if your partner or carer gives the baby a bottle of formula because they think the baby isn't getting enough breast milk, it can make breastfeeding even harder – by reducing the amount the baby wants to feed at the breast, which in turn reduces milk production.

Be guided by your baby

Babies know their own appetite. They cry when they are hungry and lose interest in feeding when they are full. You can't force a baby to breastfeed for a set amount of time or to finish a bottle. As we've seen, you need to work with your baby to maintain their ability to recognise their hunger and fullness cues.

Overly strict feeding doesn't work for older children and it doesn't work for babies either. Even babies can sense when restrictions are tight

INTRODUCE YOUR BABY TO A RANGE OF TEXTURES AND TASTES FROM ABOUT SIX MONTHS

Fussy eating

Mina and Steve were both fussy eaters when they were children and were determined to prevent their daughter Kelly, who was approaching the 'terrible twos', from going the same way.

By being good food role models Mina and Steve helped their daughter avoid the food fears that often lead to fussy eating. Steve liked making stir fries but tended to stick to chicken-based dishes. By expanding his repertoire to include fish and seafood and lots of different vegetables, he made meal times more varied and Kelly liked watching him stir everything up in the wok and was happy to try whatever he cooked. To get Kelly interested in dairy foods, Mina gave her a small pot of yoghurt for her afternoon snack every day – it's something Mina enjoys too, so they sat and ate together. Both parents are convinced these strategies have encouraged Kelly to try new foods as well as helping her avoid becoming a fussy eater.

toddlers & young children

Being a food role model for toddlers and young children

Toddlers and young children are highly impressionable – and they want to be like their parents in every way.

Family meals

Toddlers and young children thrive on family meals that offer them the chance to practise social skills and develop bonds. Sit-down meals at the table without tv and other distractions encourage conversation. They also help children to focus on what they are eating, to eat slowly and to pay attention to their body's hunger and fullness signals. Research shows that children who enjoy meals with their family, especially at dinner time, tend to have a more nutritious diet with fewer calories.

Trying new foods

Young children are naturally neophobic – they avoid new things. One of the most obvious examples is new foods. A young child will typically say an emphatic 'No' when offered something new to eat. This can lead to a child being labelled as a fussy eater and may mean that the family adapts to the child's food preferences just to avoid arguments at meal times.

In fact all children, left to their own devices, have the potential to become fussy eaters. But the way you introduce new foods can reduce the effect. Research has shown that you may have to offer a new food 10 to 14 times before your

JUST CHANGE ONE THING

Don't give in. Despite our best efforts to focus on wholesome nutritious foods, young children and toddlers soon discover that they like treats and start to ask for more. But you need to stick to the rules you've decided on for your family. Research has shown that giving treats in an irregular or unpredictable pattern reinforces children's preference for them. This is true even if you are an impeccable role model and never eat the sort of treats your children like. Conversely, rigid restrictions or avoiding treats completely doesn't work either. The best strategy to follow is to include your child's favourite treats, to teach them that treats can have a place in a healthy diet.

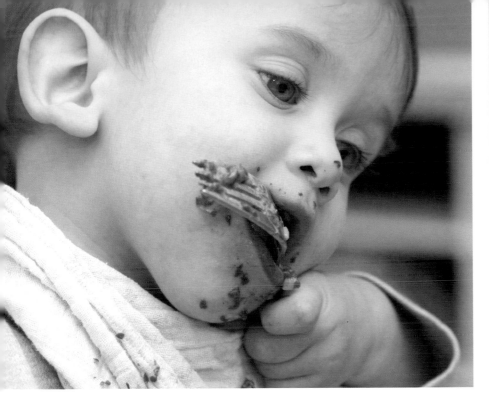

child will even taste it. So a useful strategy is to serve and eat the same foods day after day, without making a big deal out if it. Just have faith in your child and in time they'll give it a go. It helps if everyone in the family is eating the same food at the same time and with a relaxed attitude. Seeing others eating a new food takes away the fear factor for a young child.

Even when they do actually try new foods, children may not like them. But don't take this as set in stone. It's worth trying again in a few months' time, as children's tastes change as they grow.

In a study that looked at how children increased the range of foods that they ate over time, the most important factor that emerged was how many different foods a child had tried before the age of four.

Let your children choose

A good strategy for meals at home is for parents to plan menus and decide which foods to serve but to allow each member of the family to choose which foods to eat and how much of them to have.

Young children who stop eating during a meal or say that they do not want to eat are probably genuinely not hungry and should not be forced to eat. Growth slows down after infancy and you may find that your children eat less food as they grow older.

Research shows that most young children eat what we parents would call just one 'good' meal every day – and that's enough for their needs. Young children may also choose to eat only one or two foods at each meal, whereas adults usually have at least three or four different foods on their plate. That's ok too. As a

How to handle snacks

Toddlers and young children need regular snacks to keep them going throughout the day. Don't forget the difference between a snack and a treat. A snack is essentially a mini-meal and should be wholesome and nutritious. Treats are foods that are high in calories and low in nutrition but taste good. Offering different foods at snack time is a good way to increase the range of new foods your child will eat. Here are some ideas to start you off:

Sticks of raw carrot, celery, cucumber and pepper

Sliced banana, segments of orange or satsuma, slices of apple, pear or pineapple, or a small bowl of chopped fruit salad

Mini-sandwiches such as cream cheese and cucumber, bagels, mini pittas or crumpets

Plain popcorn

Cubes of cheese

Small pot of yoghurt or fromage frais

Battling over vegetables

Diane was worried that her young toddler Sam might be missing vital nutrients because he refused to eat vegetables and she was growing tired of the daily battles over broccoli and carrots.

Many parents don't realise that fruit supplies many of the same nutrients and health benefits as vegetables. Sam enjoyed fruit so Diane stopped worrying about veg and put a wide variety of fruit on the table each day. Meal times became less stressful as they stopped battling over the broccoli and gradually she was able to re-introduce vegetables with very little fuss and bother.

parent you can show your child that it's right to stop eating when you are full by sometimes leaving food on your plate too.

While meals that provide wholesome nutritious foods are a key ingredient in creating a healthy-weight home, forcing a child to eat a specific food or a specific amount of food is not helpful. It's not good for parent-child relationships and sets up mealtimes as a battleground. Attempting to be a role model by eating foods that you dislike is also unlikely to be a successful strategy.

Being a food provider for toddlers and young children

At this stage in your child's life, eating behaviour becomes as important as the actual food they put in their mouth.

Make mealtimes relaxing

As toddlers and young children learn to become independent, one of the easiest ways for them to do this is by making demands about food. Deciding whether to eat or not is one of the few things a young child can control.

The best way to deal with a child who is fussy, picky or cranky about food is to show no reaction at all to demands or tantrums. If a child

can't get a reaction, sooner or later the behaviour is abandoned. As parents we can help our children by keeping emotions separate from eating.

Children tend to be more positive about trying new foods when they are calm. Quiet meal times help young children to relax. If you're introducing a new food to a young child, make sure the whole family has some – with strict instructions that there are to be no negative words or body language to influence the youngest members. This helps young children overcome their natural fear factor.

Keep trying

Young children are often faddy about food – liking something one day, not so keen the next. So it helps to continue offering new foods, even if they were rejected before. Many of us parents make the mistake of thinking that our child hates a food just because they rejected it once. With time and exposure, and as their palate develops, young children are likely to enjoy the majority of foods we give them.

Research shows that a typical fussy eater can be described as a slime-o-phobe who doesn't like wet slimy greens. In general, fussy eaters also don't like mixed foods, with lots of different ingredients

YOUNG CHILDREN
ARE OFTEN FADDY
ABOUT FOOD, LIKING
SOMETHING ONE DAY,
THEN NOT SO KEEN
THE NEXT DAY

combined together. Separating foods out and offering them individually will get round this particular problem.

Portion sizes

If your child is already overweight, you might prefer to start off by serving smaller portions, but giving them second helpings if they ask for more. Getting them to eat slowly, focusing on taste and texture can help; as can serving lots of vegetables, fruit, vegetable soups, salads and foods that are relatively low in calories yet still help to fill you up.

Young children can be gently guided towards eating suitable portions. Questions such as, 'Does your tummy feel really full?' or 'Does your tummy feel empty?' will prompt a child to stop eating for a moment and think about hunger levels.

Treats are important too. Giving children their favourite treats, rather than just deciding for them, makes them feel empowered – and they will get even more pleasure from the treat because they chose it.

What if my child won't eat?

Children who stop eating after a few bites or skip a meal completely need a gentle reminder that there will be no more food available until the next meal or snack time. The idea is to find out whether they are full up or just not paying attention. If they insist they're not hungry, that's fine – don't encourage them to continue eating when they're not hungry. But be consistent and don't give them anything else to

Changing treats

Sunita wanted to change the type of treats she kept in the kitchen cupboard, to cut down on biscuits and sweets and focus more on wholesome nutritious food. She wondered how her children would react to the changeover and whether there would be any arguments.

On the whole, young children adapt to changes without too many awkward questions. Rather than draw attention to new additions like wholegrain cereal bars and dried fruit bars, it's best to simply include them in family meals and snacks so that they become part of the daily routine. When the children did occasionally ask if they could have a biscuit, Sunita's response was to say: 'We haven't got any right now, how about a cereal bar instead?' which was accepted without too much fuss.

JUST CHANGE ONE THING

Don't use a child's favourite foods as a reward – or take them away as a punishment. This is a common tactic to get children to behave, but it's not helpful in a healthy-weight home. Rewarding healthy eating with treats – 'eat up all your sprouts and you can have some ice cream' – teaches children that certain foods are more desirable than others. Making dessert conditional on a child having eaten all the vegetables on their plate sends the message that dessert is better than vegetables.

Damage limitation strategies

Julie wanted to limit the amount of treats she kept in the house but wasn't looking forward to her children nagging her to buy more.

Lots of parents prefer to go shopping without their children for that very reason and it's a good strategy to follow – and practical when your children are at preschool or school. And if you stock up on healthy options to offer the children instead – fun-size apples and bananas, grapes, carrot sticks, cereal bars – you're being a food enforcer for your healthy-weight home.

eat until the next family meal or snack. Children won't starve by missing a meal or two and they learn a valuable lesson. Giving in to a child's demands after they've missed a meal or refused food weakens the foundations of a healthy-weight home.

Many children have a built-in preference for foods that are high in fat and calories. Because the calories in these foods are highly concentrated, it's easy to eat too many. Keep these foods for treats. Giving in to preferences isn't helpful – and neither is using food as a reward. Giving food as a reward makes that food seem special and makes it even more desirable.

We should give both familiar and new foods to our children

with very little fuss. Toddlers and young children tend to accept what they're given as long as they have no reason to suspect the foods are different. Drawing attention to a food swap, for example, by announcing that you are replacing semi-skimmed milk with skimmed milk, can lead to the children rejecting the change. So keep any changes low-key.

You can always improve on tradition

All ethnic heritages and cultures include wholesome nutritious foods, making the 5 Simple Rules easy to incorporate into every family. There is no need to abandon traditional foods to create a healthy-weight home.

JUST CHANGE ONE THING

Let your child decide how much they want to eat. Presenting a child with a 'plated' meal is bound to cause tensions when a child disagrees with how much you wish them to eat. The easier option is to put dishes of food on the table and get them to help themselves, rather than ask them how much they want of each item when you are serving up. As a parent it can feel quite scary to allow your child to decide how much food they want on their plate. But research on preschool children has shown that children who were allowed to respond to their own hunger and fullness signals had a fairly steady calorie intake over the course of the study. Encouraging children to decide how much to eat helps them to balance the calories they are taking in with the calories their bodies are using up. The focus on wholesome nutritious foods in a healthy-weight home makes it less likely that children will overeat.

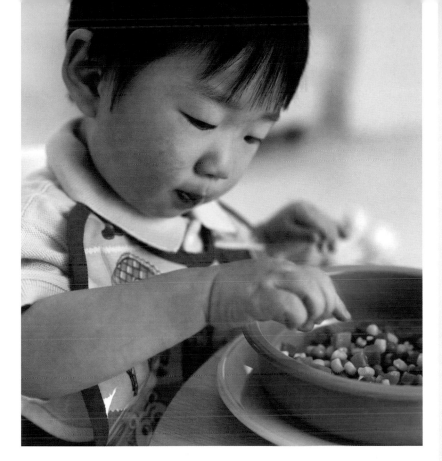

Some parents can feel at a disadvantage in trying to create a healthy-weight home because the traditional dishes that they cook seem to tick all the wrong boxes in terms of healthy eating.

But no matter what your style of cooking there are always simple changes you can make to your recipes that will create more wholesome and nutritious meals. What's more, the family is unlikely even to notice the difference.

Examples include substituting brown rice for white – try serving a mixture of the two at first – and reducing the amount of oil you use in recipes by switching to a cooking-oil spray. You can also research recipes that use a wider range of vegetables.

Being a food enforcer for toddlers and young children

Many toddlers and young children can seem downright difficult. Saying no, refusing to eat and defying grown-ups is what they do best.

What's normal?

Understanding that this difficult behaviour is part of normal development helps us to deal with it – as does coming up with new strategies and approaches to enforce healthy eating.

Young children respond well when food rules are enforced gently but firmly. The enforcer tells the child what the choices are, allows the child to choose and

The toddler who didn't know when to stop

Louise and Chris couldn't believe how much their son Freddie ate. He'd had a big appetite since he was a baby and if they didn't stop him, he wouldn't stop eating of his own accord.

In our role as food providers we need to serve our children appropriate-size portions. Louise and Chris began by giving Freddie smaller portions and if he asked for second helpings, they only gave him a little more. By asking him whether he felt full, they got him to think about his feelings of hunger and begin to recognise the signs of being full up. To take his mind off food, they encouraged him to go off to play after dinner but said he could always come back for more food if he still felt hungry. He rarely did return to the table once he got absorbed in an interesting game.

Snack or treat?

Jo's children Luke and Ben were confused. When they went to play with their friends, they were offered biscuits or crisps as a snack, but at home a snack was fruit or cheese and crackers.

The best way to explain the difference between a snack and a treat in a healthy-weight home is to tell children that a snack is an 'anytime' food that can be eaten whenever they are hungry. Jo told Ben and Luke that many of the foods they are offered at friends' houses are really treats and she explained that treats are fine but they are not foods that you can eat all the time – then the boys understood what was going on.

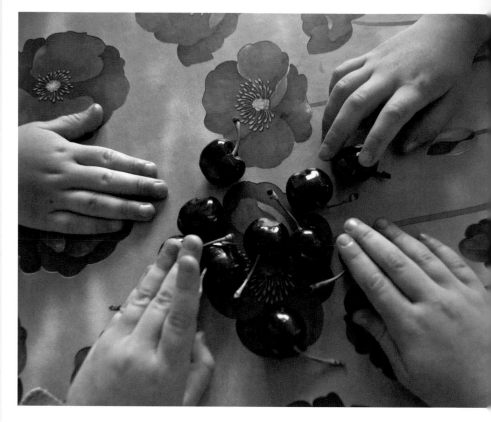

does not react emotionally if the child says no or has a tantrum. We all know how hard it can be to avoid reacting but a calm approach signals that you are in charge and that emotional outbursts are not going to change your mind.

Eating greens is a common battleground between youngsters and adults, and encouraging a child to enjoy vegetables takes a lot of effort. Children naturally prefer sweet foods, so aren't keen on the strong flavours of some vegetables. Vegetables need to be part of daily meals, and by calmly including the same ones several meals in

succession, without making a big deal about it, we can overcome a child's natural resistance. Seeing the rest of the family eating vegetables always helps.

Snacks are important

Young children need snacks – their stomachs are too small to hold enough food to keep them going from just three meals a day. Think of a snack as a mini-meal and give children the same foods they have at mealtimes, such as cereal, fruit or a small sandwich. This helps children learn the vital difference between a snack and a treat.

Managing family meals

Including toddlers and young children in family meals sets the foundation for family eating habits for years to come. It's also an ideal opportunity for young children to see how other members of the family eat.

Research has shown that children are more likely to eat fruit and vegetables if they see others doing the same – especially if they get used to this by late infancy. Young children's natural fear of anything new is reduced when new foods are seen as a natural part of a family meal.

A positive approach to occasional treats

Being overly strict about treats can result in a child becoming obsessed with them, and the child may overeat if offered treats at a friend's house. Toddlers and young children don't cope very well with absolute restrictions, so at the very least, try setting a family policy that says, 'We don't serve these foods at home but it's ok to eat them when visiting friends.'

Enforcing doesn't mean putting a child on a diet

Experts are against dieting for young children. And it's never a good idea to comment on a young child's weight or body shape. In a study of young girls, the girls who gained the most weight were those who were on a strict diet and who were worried about their weight and body shape.

In our role as food enforcers, we need to look for alternatives to dieting – especially by focusing on wholesome nutritious foods that promote a healthy weight.

Don't be too strict

Kevin has two young children: Lewis, who is six months old and Lily, age three. Lily didn't have any sugary foods until she was one year old, but two years later she is now very keen on sweets. Kevin wondered whether he should be as strict with Lewis, since restricting Lily's sugar intake when she was small doesn't seem to have had a lasting effect on her preference for sweet things.
Being too rigid with rules doesn't always have the desired effect. Kevin may well have been so strict with Lily that she reacted by wanting and enjoying sweet foods even more as a result. He decided to be less strict with his son. It would be difficult to restrict Lewis's sugar intake in the same way in any case since he will see his sister eating treats.

JUST CHANGE ONE THING

Children who are old enough to use a spoon can actually feed themselves, so let them do it. We're often reluctant to let children have a go because they take so long and make such a mess. But we have to see past the hassle and think of the benefits. Not only does letting children feed themselves encourage physical skills and coordination, it helps them to know their limits and get the calories their bodies need without overeating. This is even more important when they are eating treats like ice cream and biscuits. Giving a child a small portion and letting them feed themselves lets them have the pleasure of eating treats without too many calories.

Treat everyone equally

John and Vicky have two teenage daughters; Harriet is at a healthy weight, but Sally could do with losing a few pounds. The parents were planning to prepare separate meals for Sally to help her manage her weight.

Isolating a family member with a weight problem in this way is rarely successful. Rule 5 (the rules apply to everyone in the home) is designed to help families avoid making this mistake. By making changes to the food everyone eats, everyone gains health benefits and the daughter with a weight problem will bring it under control. John and Vicky started buying skimmed milk instead of full-fat, served water with meals rather than soft drinks and used a cooking-oil spray to reduce the amount of oil they cooked with. They barely noticed these simple changes but all of them soon began to appreciate the difference they made.

older children

Being a food role model for older children

Older children spend more time away from home and become more independent in their food choices. Many buy snacks and occasional meals for themselves. Even so, parents are still a big influence on their eating habits.

Family meals

Eating together as a family sends out an important message to older children: they learn the value of sitting down and eating with their parents and siblings no matter how busy the family schedule. And as parents, we are being role models and showing that family meals are part of daily life. A relaxed dinner-table atmosphere can help older children unwind and open up about what's going on in their lives. Family traditions such as Sunday lunch, Saturday morning family breakfast and special occasion meals all enhance the joy of eating.

It's still the parents' responsibility to decide what foods to cook and when to eat. But older children should be encouraged to serve themselves and decide how much to eat. Research shows that children who help themselves tend to take smaller portions.

With their parents on hand as positive food role models, older children may begin to realise that eating a lot of treats such as chips, crisps, sweets, biscuits and soft drinks can lead to excess weight; at the same time they'll discover that focusing on wholesome nutritious foods can help them manage their weight.

JUST CHANGE ONE THING

Stop snacking while you watch tv. Your children are guaranteed to follow your example and do exactly the same. Older children who nibble and watch tv may not even be fully aware of what and how much they have eaten. It can be a hard habit to break, especially when children have just got in from school. Limiting screen time and, if possible, having a house rule of not eating in front of the tv (set goals as mentioned earlier) are good strategies for the entire family.

Being a food role model outside the home

As parents we need to carry on being a food role model when we go out to eat as well as when we are at home. Older children in particular watch how their parents make food choices when the family is eating out. Research has shown that super-sized meals and large portions encourage children to eat more. In one study, children served a double-size portion took larger bites and ate more calories. If parents themselves go ahead and order extra-large portions it sends the message to their children that this amount of food is appropriate.

Once older children can read and understand the information on menus, you can discuss what's on offer and what they have chosen. Although you can't control what teenagers eat when they go out with friends, making sure they are informed about nutrition will help them to make good food choices independently.

Comfort food

When children see parents use food to cheer themselves up they learn that food can be a powerful coping mechanism. They also learn to eat between meals and to have a snack if they feel stressed. However, seeing parents who have learned to handle stress and

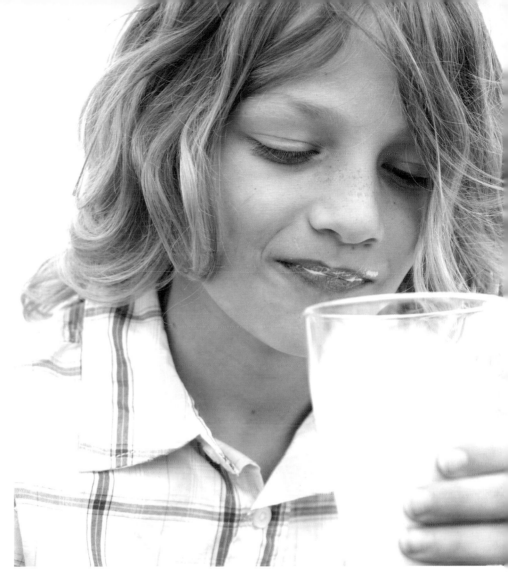

emotional ups and downs using other methods, including physical activity, private time and non-food rewards, helps children learn vital coping skills – an important factor in lasting weight management.

A RELAXED DINNER TABLE CAN HELP OLDER CHILDREN UNWIND AND OPEN UP ABOUT WHAT'S GOING ON IN THEIR LIVES

Traffic lights make shopping easy

When you're staring at the foods on the supermarket shelves, how can you be sure you're choosing the healthiest option? Many manufacturers and supermarkets now use 'traffic light' labelling to help you decide. These show you at a glance whether a product is high in fats, saturated fats, sugar and salt. A red 'light' on the front of a packet means you might want to eat this food occasionally as a treat; amber means it's neither high or low in that particular ingredient but you may need to keep an eye on levels; while green means go right ahead, this is a healthy choice. Most products will have a mixture of all three colours. If you're in a real hurry, it's simple – just go for as many greens as possible. If you have time to stop and read the labels you can make a more informed choice. Although the design of the labels varies between brands, you can compare them with complete confidence as all manufacturers use the same guidelines. Visit www.eatwell.gov.uk and click on Food Labels for more information.

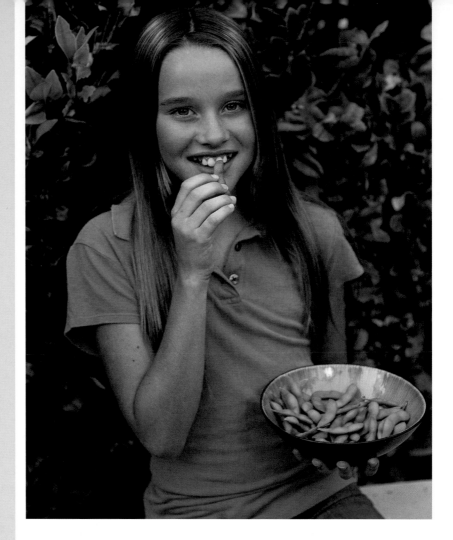

	low per 100g **GREEN**	medium per 100g **AMBER**	high per 100g RED
Fat	0 - 3g	3g - 20g	20g and over
Saturated fat	0 - 1.5g	1.5 - 5g	5g and over
Total sugars	0 - 5g	5g - 15g	15g and over
Salt	0.03g	0.3 - 1.5g	1.5g and over

Being a food provider for older children

Older children are both harder and easier to deal with than younger ones. Although they are able to understand how their food choices affect their weight, rebellious adolescents may not want to follow the 5 Simple Rules.

Have faith

Experts recommend that in these situations parents carry on as normal providing wholesome nutritious meals, even if their efforts are undermined by teenagers eating out, bringing

TEENAGERS OFTEN RAID THE FRIDGE: TAKE ADVANTAGE OF THIS AND STOCK IT WITH WHOLESOME NUTRITIOUS FOODS

home extra treats or missing meals. As parents we need to have faith in ourselves and believe that we are doing the right thing. Often the lessons that are learned as a young child but then rejected as a teenager do return later on in young adulthood.

Carry on introducing new foods at mealtimes. As children enter their preteens they may be willing to try new foods, even if they're not so keen on some of them. This is quite different from younger children, who tend not to want to try any new foods once they've tasted something they don't like.

Teenagers often hang out in the kitchen, raiding the fridge and eating whatever is on offer. Take advantage of this by stocking up on wholesome nutritious foods. Research shows that when these foods are readily available for children to help themselves, they will eat more of them. At the same time, it's a good idea to limit the quantities of sugary soft drinks you keep in the house, as these have been linked to increased weight gain and higher BMI.

Mixed messages

Children who are not allowed to eat when they are truly hungry get the message that they should eat when food is around instead of when they're hungry, which isn't a good idea. This doesn't mean that you should hand out food when a child has missed a meal through choice. True hunger takes many hours to develop and the likelihood of a child reaching a harmful level of hunger between family meals and snacks in a typical home is virtually nil.

In homes where there are extreme food rules children may eat even when they are not hungry. Research has shown that mothers who restrict what they themselves eat, combined with times when they are out of control around food, tend to restrict their daughters' food intake, who then become prone to overeating and gaining weight. Being too authoritarian in our role as food provider reduces our chances of creating a healthy-weight home. Children respond best to providers who are consistent, firm and supportive.

Being a food enforcer for older children

Until they reach their rebellious teens, older children are proof that enforcing the 5 Simple Rules really does pay off. Most eat a good variety of foods at this age.

What's typical?

Older children still need regular family mealtimes. Although they may have quite a busy social life by now, enforcing regular meals

New ways to celebrate

Dave was concerned that Easter had become an excuse to indulge in far too much chocolate – not to mention a blow-out roast dinner with the grandparents. His children Connor and Emma are aged 10 and 12, so he thought they should be old enough to sit down and talk about how their traditional Easter didn't really fit in with the idea of a healthy-weight home.

Looking for new ways to celebrate a family tradition can be a positive way of continuing to mark special occasions. Dave, Connor and Emma decided to turn Easter Sunday into an outing instead. They packed a picnic and cycled to a nearby forest trail and made their own Easter egg treasure hunt. They still had plenty of treats but they were a lot more active than they normally were on Easter Sunday. And to make sure the children's grandparents didn't feel left out, they cycled over to see them on their way home.

Getting to grips with portion size

Clive and Ellen's three sons were starting to gain too much weight and their parents realised that the boys had no idea what a reasonable portion size was. They were also too fond of chips and ready meals.

Food packaging contains helpful information on portion sizes and nutrition and is a good way to get an idea of what you're eating. Boys also tend to respond well to learning from a male role model, so Clive got the boys interested in studying the nutritional information on their favourite ready meals. He told them about the Traffic Lights System (see page 96 for more information), which gives guidance on the fat, sugar and salt content of foods. And they also discussed appropriate portion sizes at meal times. The boys became enthusiastic converts and soon started scrutinising what Clive and Ellen were eating and telling them how they could improve some of their food choices.

PLANNING AHEAD MAKES THE JOB OF BEING A FOOD ENFORCER A LOT EASIER, ESPECIALLY WHEN TIME IS TIGHT

is essential. Older children will be confident in their own ability to choose wholesome foods, and family meal times give you the chance to build on this by congratulating them on their good sense. Research has also shown that family meals improve older children's general health and well-being, not just how well-nourished they are. Children who eat with their family are less likely to take up smoking, drinking alcohol or using drugs. They're also less likely to become depressed.

Teenagers who sit down to eat with the family regularly learn to appreciate that family meals are important. And if family meals are mostly happy relaxing times, then teenagers are less likely to develop eating disorders. Research has shown that making time for family meals – even when life is extremely hectic – is the single most important thing that protects girls against eating disorders, and also deters them from following fad diets to lose weight. With older children it's even more important to ban any comments on their weight. Keep the focus on a healthy lifestyle instead.

Planning ahead

Consistency is a key part of being a food enforcer and many parents find planning ahead makes the job a whole lot easier. Examples include keeping bottled water and snacks in the car so there's no excuse to stop at the shop on the way home from school or after football practice. Cooking and freezing meals at the weekend saves time during the week, as does starting dinner off before work in the slow cooker or buying ready-prepared veg and meat – all strategies that will help you

JUST CHANGE ONE THING

Be a consistent food provider for everyone in the family. When overweight children are given different food and different rules from those family members at a healthy weight, their confidence and self esteem can be affected – and they're likely to feel deprived. This is one of the main reasons why the 5 Simple Rules apply to everyone.

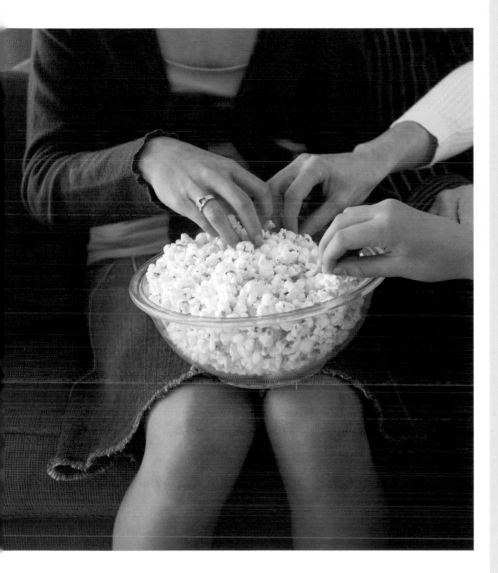

Making the right choice from the menu

Lizzie's son James was captain of the under-15s football team and doing really well. Because practice ended so late on Fridays, when she picked him up she took him to a burger bar straight afterwards. Although she was very proud of how active James was, at the same time she worried about what he chose to eat when they were out.

This is where being a food role model comes in. Over time Lizzie influenced her son's choice by consistently making healthy nutritious choices herself. Week after week Lizzie ordered grilled chicken and salad with low-fat dressing or a baked potato with a low-fat filling like baked beans or tuna. Much to her surprise, after a while James started to choose similar foods. He didn't do it all the time but Lizzie was reassured that he was getting the message – and all without any arguments.

achieve your goal of serving up wholesome meals during the week.

Teens and family meals

Family meals are good for teenage girls, not just nutritionally but for their emotional health and well-being too. One way to get teens back to the dinner table – girls and boys – is to encourage them to cook every now and then. If they are not very confident at first, get them to try putting together no-cook ingredients like dips and pitta breads and salads for everyone to help themselves. Once they've got that under their belt they can progress to simple recipes. Appreciation from the rest of the family will boost their confidence.

active parents, active children

One of the most fundamental changes to our lifestyles over the decades has been the drop in activity levels. Now we're less inclined to walk anywhere when we can drive, and our homes are full of labour-saving equipment that reduces how physically active we are. The human body just wasn't designed to spend hours at a desk or sitting on the sofa – and we suffer accordingly when we do. And we're passing these habits on to the next generation.

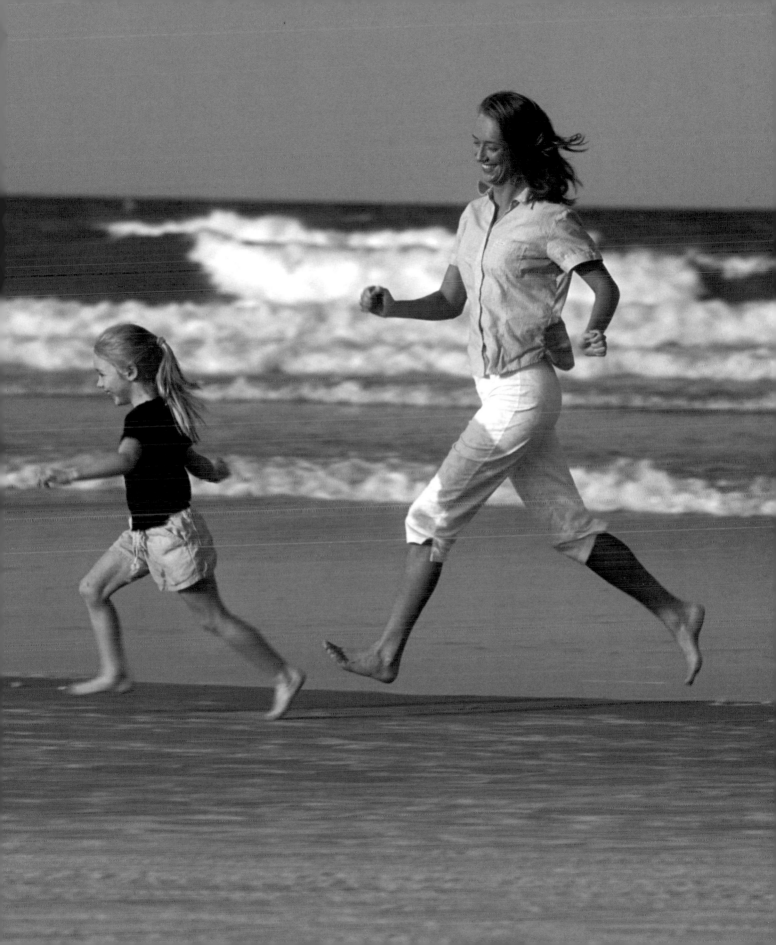

Good activity role models
➔ are active people
➔ take part in structured exercise as well as being active in general
➔ limit the amount of time they spend watching tv
➔ plan family outings that include activity
➔ are active for at least 60 minutes a day

How much activity?

Recommended levels of activity are 30 minutes a day of moderately intense activity – such as brisk walking, cycling or walking up stairs – at least five days a week. In a survey for the Department of Health in 2004, just 35% of men and 24% of women interviewed achieved these levels. Children tend to do better. In 2005 and 2006, 80% of school children did two hours or more PE and sports a week, which is still below the target for a healthy-weight home but is heading in the right direction. The government has set a new target for schools to ensure that pupils have access to at least five hours of PE and sport each week, and outside school, children will benefit from investment in updating 3,500 playgrounds across the country.

HOW TO BE AN ACTIVITY ROLE MODEL

Children need positive activity role models, both at home and in the outside world. As parents we are their primary role models. Children learn by watching how we spend our free time – from going for a walk, to going to the gym once a week, to how much tv we watch.

To be a positive activity role model you need to look for ways to make movement a part of your day. A good starting point is to be

JUST CHANGE ONE THING

If you head for the escalator or lift in department stores – stop. Walk up the stairs instead, and do the same at work.

aware of lots of small opportunities to be more active. For example, when you go shopping, park in the carpark furthest from the shops so you have to walk a bit further – get a wheelie shopper to make it easier. Take the dog for an extra walk – he'll be grateful and you'll benefit too. Don't jump in the car just to post a letter or buy a loaf of bread – walk instead. If you haven't got acres of grass, using a push mower rather than an electric or petrol version is a great way to get exercise. In autumn try raking up leaves instead.

Activity role models also enjoy planned exercise at the gym or badminton club, yoga or Pilates classes, golf, tennis – whatever's available locally.

Limiting the amount of time spent passively in front of a screen – whether it's the tv or the computer or even texting on your mobile – is one of the 5 Simple Rules for a healthy-weight home. If your children see you reducing the time you spend watching tv, they'll soon get the message.

How much time do I need to spend on exercise?

30 minutes a day of moderately intense activity – such as walking briskly, not just ambling along – helps lower blood pressure and reduce stress levels. But while 30 minutes a day has definite health benefits, it's not enough to maintain your weight if you've already lost a few pounds, and neither is it enough to help you lose weight. In a healthy-weight home 60 minutes of activity is ideal – for all adults who don't want to gain weight and for all children regardless of their weight. Adults who have lost weight may need to aim for 90 minutes a day to maintain their new weight.

How will I find the time?

In today's busy lifestyles squeezing in an extra hour's activity for ourselves and the children can seem an impossible goal. The good news is that the recommended activity levels are based on cumulative activity – that is, lots of small activities added together. You'll find that plenty of everyday activities you already do will count towards your daily total – for example, walking the dog, hanging out the washing, running around with your children at the park. Make the most of these opportunities throughout the day

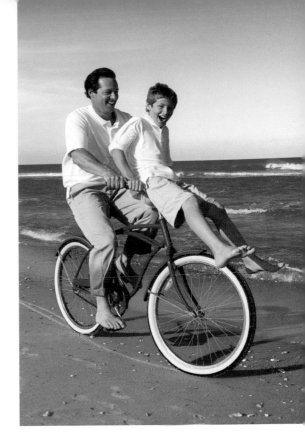

and the minutes quickly add up. Include a few structured sports or activities during the week, and you're there. How many minutes or hours have you achieved today?

Think of the benefits

Being active is one of the best things that a family can do – you'll benefit more from increasing your family's activity levels than just about any other lifestyle change you can make. And one of the key benefits is being able to control your weight. Research has shown lack of physical activity is one of the major factors when children are overweight, and activity helps prevent a child from developing weight problems in the first place.

Regular physical activity also builds muscles and boosts the body's metabolism, and reduces a child's body fat levels. It helps children to build strong bones – and may reduce the chances of them having weak bones as adults. Active adults reduce their chances of developing heart disease, diabetes and certain cancers.

One of the best side effects is that being active makes you feel better straight away – it improves your mood and cheers you up.

Start slowly

As with most lifestyle changes, it's best to start off gradually. Taking

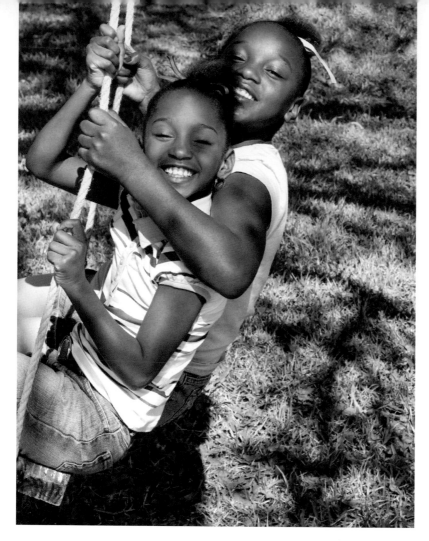

coordinating the development of cycling across the country) is planning to improve cycle routes and provide more cycling training to children. Schools are being encouraged to develop a travel plan to persuade pupils to cycle to school where practical. Since the early 1990s there's been a steady increase in the number of children going to school by car rather than walking or cycling. The number of children aged between five and 10 years old who walk to school decreased from 61% in 1992-4 to 52% in 2002-3.

Prove it yourself

As active parents we can inspire our children to be active too. We can show them that activity is important and worth the time and effort – and prove that it is possible to fit activity into a busy day. Research shows that children are more likely to take part in an activity that their parents enjoy too. Children also feel particularly good about being active when they get lots of encouragement from their family.

Combined with a shift towards wholesome nutritious foods, regular activity affects the 'calories in, calories out' balance that we talked about in Chapter 3 – helping stop weight gain and helping children grow into their weight.

small steps in the right direction, first to be more active in daily life and then increasing the amount of structured exercise or sport you do, is more likely to be successful than rushing into major changes. This sort of approach is good for children – it helps them develop patterns that will stay with them for life.

Take up cycling

Many children fall short of Rule 4 (60 minutes of activity a day) and we need to look at ways of working more activity into their day. Cycling England (the national body for

BEING AN ACTIVITY PROVIDER

To be an effective activity provider the best thing you can do is make sure your children have plenty of opportunities to be active. Children have naturally high energy levels – something we often envy. They love to run around and have fun. In fact, most children will be active without being told to. Though sometimes they need a bit of help to inspire their natural instincts and you might need a few ideas on how to go about it.

When getting children on the move, you've got the choice between unstructured activities like playing in the garden or going for a bike ride, and organised activities like team sports. Organised sports can mean re-jigging the family's schedule on certain days to fit in clubs and matches, so you'll need to show commitment.

Help out in any way you can

As an activity provider you can give your children a helping hand simply by inviting friends round to play. You can provide outdoor toys and sports equipment, and lifts to sports clubs and matches. You can take your commitment even further and volunteer to be a coach or a referee for the local football team, say, or just offer to help out in any way you can, by giving other players a lift or helping with half-time refreshments.

Praising your child's efforts can be a big help in motivating them. Many children are naturally reluctant to try an activity without a gentle push. Showing interest and recognising achievements when they've made progress – or being sympathetic when things haven't gone according to plan – and offering useful suggestions for improvement, are all part of being an activity provider.

Believe in your children

It's actually been proved that children whose parents believe in their ability to perform are more likely to take up an activity that is physically challenging. Having confidence in your children – and supporting them in whatever they choose to do – in turn creates confident children who have faith in their own physical skills and have a positive attitude towards their achievements.

The activity providers – who are typically mum and dad – create a healthy-weight home by encouraging daily activity and making it as easy as possible. Regular activity is so important that it is one of the 5 Simple Rules. And a home environment that embraces activity as part of daily life will inspire active children.

Good activity providers supply
→ sports equipment and toys
→ opportunities
→ encouragement
→ support
→ praise
→ motivation
→ feedback
→ reinforcement

Your action plan for activity
→ Investigate what's available at your local leisure centre
→ Choose something that the whole family wants to do, e.g. ice skating, roller skating or blading, indoor rock climbing, swimming
→ Work out which evenings are best for family activities or set aside a regular time at the weekend

Make it fun

If you make fun the main aim of being active it's almost guaranteed that children will want to be part of the action. Experts agree that young children should not be forced to exercise as a way of losing weight and many teenagers would rebel against being told to do so. By focusing on fun, you take away the potential for activity to become a chore or a drag. In a healthy-weight home activities are enjoyable, rewarding and part of the family lifestyle – any health and weight benefits are a bonus.

The fun factor of any activity goes up once children are confident in their ability. A trip to the ice rink is a lot more fun once they can whizz round without falling over – and leave their flailing parents far behind. There are so many challenging activities out there – from dry ski slopes to snowboarding to indoor rock-climbing in the heart of the city – and leisure centres are only too keen to offer taster courses and introductory sessions.

BEING AN ACTIVITY ENFORCER

An activity enforcer makes sure everyone in the home is active – it's that simple.

When we look back at our own childhood we remember setting off on bike rides that lasted all day, building camps in the woods, family games of cricket on the beach. Children today have far more options for entertainment and aren't so reliant on creating their own fun. And very often it's not practical to try to recreate those nostalgic pastimes, especially with more traffic on the roads and fewer places to play that haven't been fenced off and surrounded with 'keep out' notices.

Instead we have to turn to more structured outings to make sure our children get enough activity; in most cases, we can't just send them out of the house and hope they'll get on with it. As a parent and activity enforcer we have to learn how to manage the family's free time. Once again there's a delicate balance between being firm and consistent, and being too strict. This is easy to say but quite another thing to put into practice. One of the best ways is to combine two roles – that of activity role model and activity enforcer. Telling your children what to do and actually doing it yourself gives you authority and credibility – your children will see you being active and not just talking about it.

Leading by example

Research has been done into the way parents make a big difference when they lead by example. Two groups of children were monitored while they were trying to change their behaviour. In one group the children were taught directly by researchers. In the second group, the researchers taught the parents what to do and they passed on their new skills to their children. The children who had been taught by their parents were more successful in changing their behaviour. This should give us all the motivation we need to get on with building activity into our lives and our children's.

How can I encourage activity?

The biggest hurdle is finding something that your child wants to do. Don't fall into the trap of thinking that if you liked playing tennis when you were young then your child is bound to too. Don't be disappointed if your child doesn't share your passion for football or ballet – help them find out what they want to do.

Often inspiration comes from a visit to watch a big football match or a dance performance – look out for special offers in your local paper for outings to matches or shows. Children who enjoy what they're doing are far more likely to stick to it.

While you need to encourage your child to choose an activity, you do need to double check their choice of sport or exercise to make sure that it is both practical and safe. For example, weight lifting is fine for adults and older teenagers but isn't recommended for young children.

The family that exercises together stays together

When all members of the family join in an activity it brings everyone closer together, as well as improving the chances that everyone sticks at it. In one study children were shown to be almost six times more likely to be active when both parents were active, compared to children whose parents had a sedentary lifestyle. Unfortunately, inactive parents have a greater influence on their children than active parents.

Active parents do not guarantee active children, but inactive parents are very unlikely to have active children.

The other bonus about family activities is that opportunities for sitting in front of the tv or computer are seriously reduced when the whole family is having fun together. That is why Rules 3 and 4 work so well together:

RULE 3: Limit screen time to a maximum of two hours a day
RULE 4: Try to be active for an hour or more every day

Winter activities

Diana and Tom and their three children were an active family who enjoyed going on bike rides, playing tennis, running and rollerblading. But in the winter their activity levels dropped.

There is plenty to do undercover in winter – swimming, ice skating, dance classes, yoga. Visit your local leisure centre or fitness centre and see what's on offer. And cycling is still fun on cold crisp days, as is a family hike.

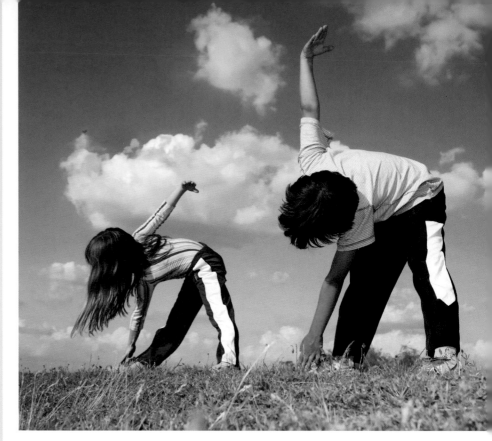

Motivating teenage boys

Paula and Joe wanted to motivate their teenage son Mark. Left to his own devices he wasn't interested in being active at all and preferred to sit in front of his computer all day.

You have to make it clear that teenagers can't opt out of being active. Paula and Joe presented Mark with a list of ideas they'd come up with and he reluctantly agreed to get his bike out of the shed. He started off riding round the block and met other boys who were heading for the playing fields. There he kicked a football around and played a bit of basketball. Now he heads off with friends most afternoons after school and has even joined the school basketball team.

Research has shown that over the course of their childhood, children who watched the most tv gained the most body fat. Another study concluded that being inactive is directly related to excess weight gain in children. That's why experts recommend limiting screen time to two hours a day. It may sound restrictive but it's based on scientific evidence. In some families it will be a hard target to achieve but it will make everyone more selective in their tv viewing or surfing the net or playing online or computer games, as well as having health benefits.

Motivation is vital

As an activity enforcer you need to motivate the family. Children with supportive parents are more likely to want to be active in the first place and will be confident of their own physical skills. Confidence is very important for strenuous activities such as skipping or jogging. As parents we can boost our children's belief in themselves – their self efficacy – by making sure they learn the basic physical skills they need, like riding a bike, hitting a ball or swimming, which will give them a good basis for all sorts of other activities. There is evidence that boys are particularly influenced by their fathers – how active they are and how much they encourage their sons.

What shall we do today?

Decisions on how to spend family free time happen daily. Creating family policies and practices that encourage activity is essential. A bit of planning can make all the difference. Use charts and lists pinned up in the kitchen to remind everyone of all the options – having a list of bad weather ideas will go some way to stopping everyone slumping in front of the tv on wet weekends. Have a noticeboard and pin up leaflets from the local pool so that you don't get caught out by not knowing opening hours, add leaflets from the leisure centre, notices of charity walks, community fun runs, etc.

Many schools re-open in the evenings to let locals use their facilities. The facilities will vary depending on whether it's a primary school or a secondary school, but you may be able to use the gym, dance studio, swimming pool or netball courts.

Get out of the house

There is a strong correlation between how much time a child spends outside and how active they are. Of course it helps to have somewhere to play and some simple equipment. If you have space in your garden, swings, a trampoline or netball hoop will make all the difference.

Public playgrounds should be part of the answer but in reality our playgrounds have been allowed to decline over the years and are often places where gangs congregate and leave litter, so they are no longer a fun family destination for parents of young children. But with government funding in place to revamp thousands of parks, they should become part of our local resources once more.

It's not just about sports and exercise

Housework uses up energy and gets you moving. It's something children can be involved in, and for the best chance of success, choose the right jobs for each child. Helping to prepare food can be a fun activity: it teaches them how to make healthy meals as well as getting them away from the tv. Try helping them to make delicious smoothies, wholemeal fruit muffins and tasty burgers.

Jobs to get children moving
→ Sweeping up – indoors and out
→ Washing the car – more fun when two people do it
→ Walking the dog
→ Vacuuming – listening to an iPod
→ Stripping the beds – do it together and sing a song
→ Cleaning the bath
→ Cleaning the downstairs windows – inside and out

Adding up the hours

Michael drove his mum Andrea to despair – he was addicted to video games and never went anywhere without his Nintendo DS. And he certainly wasn't active for an hour a day.

Rule 3 limits screen time to two hours a day maximum. As Michael liked to spend longer than that in one session Andrea came up with the idea of letting him 'bank' some of his hours during the week so he could spend more time playing at the weekend. With the extra free time created on weekdays Andrea encouraged him to go out on his bike or hit a tennis ball in the garden. At first Michael kept a close eye on how many hours he'd accumulated but as time went by he stopped being so concerned and actually started taking a football on family outings instead of his DS.

Ideal first toys for active babies
→ Play mat with different textures
→ A rattle that is easy to grip
→ Simple cloth toy
→ Safety baby mirror that can be propped in the cot or attached to the pram
→ Baby gym with interesting dangly toys

babies

Being an activity role model for babies

Babies aren't really very active for the first six months or so. But they still take notice of what's happening around them. Physical skills begin to develop in infancy and are boosted by the toys babies have to play with, their surroundings and the way we interact with them. Colourful mobiles to look at, music to listen to and lots of playtime with everyone in the family help babies learn how to move and explore their world.

A good way to start is by making eye contact with your baby and once you've got their attention, smile, pull faces, stick your tongue out and get them to respond. Your baby will also enjoy lying on a mat on the floor so that they can kick their legs and move their arms freely. Leave your baby's feet bare when it's warm enough and they'll have lots of fun playing with their toes.

As they get older a baby swing or baby walker or bouncer can keep a baby amused, but keep an eye on how much time they spend in them. While it may look like a baby is having plenty of fun in a walker or bouncer, it can actually restrict the way a baby moves.

Older babies enjoy playing in the bath – with you there at all times, of course – so look out for colourful bath toys. Simple cups, sponges, sieves and funnels for pouring water will encourage active play.

Chewy toys that are easy to hold and are designed to be put in the mouth are a good idea at this age. Activity centres with things to press or twist can be attached to the bars of a cot.

When your baby can sit up – from six to 12 months – they'll enjoy rolling a ball to you. And once they've learned to crawl they will probably race after it themselves. Building bricks – wooden or plastic – will get them to practise hand-eye coordination.

Being an activity provider for babies

Let's face it, until they begin to crawl, babies can't get very far on their own, so they rely on parents and childminders to make sure they get the activity they need. They need encouragement to move their arms and legs, to practise reaching and grabbing, and later on to try standing and learning to walk.

Babies need anything from 30

minutes to an hour's playtime a day, but not necessarily all in one session – most babies can't play for an hour without getting tired. And they can't usually play by themselves – get family members to join in with games of peek a boo, hide the teddy, roll the ball.

Babies need a safe place to play, such as a blanket or playmat on the floor. As they start to move you'll have to keep an eye on the environment: look out for sharp furniture edges, fit safety covers to electric sockets, put child locks on cupboards. While it may seem like a safe option, leaving a baby in a cot, playpen or pram for a long time doesn't provide them with a stimulating environment.

Being an activity enforcer for babies

Babies can't be active on their own; they need activity built into their daily routine. If your baby spends time with a childminder, it's important to discuss this with them. Be clear about what you want to happen and give childminders proper instructions – don't be vague or you may end up disappointed. Tell your childminder that you don't want your baby to spend a lot of time in a pram, cot or high chair. Find out in advance how they keep their small charges amused – do they have a baby gym? A playpen?

Activity helps babies develop the muscles and skills they are going to need to learn to sit, stand and walk. Babies who spend a lot of time confined in a high chair, push chair or pram miss out on vital chances to build these skills. Long periods of inactivity means that babies aren't getting the message that movement has to be an important part of each day.

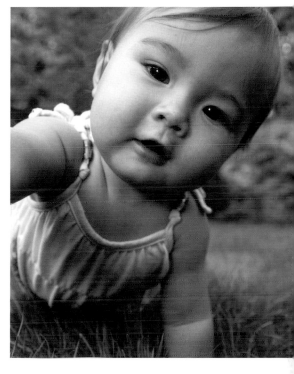

Toys that encourage babies to move
➔ Push along trolleys for when they're ready to practise standing
➔ Different size balls
➔ Bricks for stacking to help coordination

JUST CHANGE ONE THING

Join a mother and toddler group. It's a great way to meet other parents and to get children socialising and playing together. Groups are typically held in a community centre, church hall or village hall, and there's usually a small weekly fee to take part. Your health visitor or your local Children's Information Service will be able to put you in touch with a group near you – or simply check the hall or community centre noticeboards or look for notices in your doctor's surgery or health centre. If there isn't a group nearby, think about setting one up. The Preschool Learning Alliance has detailed advice on its website www.pre-school.org.uk/baby-and-toddler/

All for one and one for all

Debbie and Richard have five school-age children. While they are working towards creating a healthy-weight home, they realised that without being aware of it, they had drifted apart as a family. They all did their own thing, and family activities had become a thing of the past – the children did various sports on an irregular basis and Debbie and Richard had got used to sitting around doing nothing.

Until all the children are teenagers and object to being seen with mum and dad, family activities are the ideal way to demonstrate that activity is a crucial element of the healthy-weight home – as well as lots of fun. Debbie realised that their lifestyle wasn't helping them manage their weight and that they were growing apart as a family so she decided to do something about it. She planned a day out at the local park and made a chart of different activities for everyone to try, including rollerblading, skateboarding and traditional racquet and ball games. They took a picnic and plenty of bottled water: the children had a really good time and begged mum to organise another day out soon.

toddlers & young children

Being an activity role model for toddlers and young children

Once toddlers start to walk, there's absolutely no stopping them. During these early years, children learn all the basic physical skills such as running, jumping, hopping, skipping, throwing and catching, kicking and balancing. Children who are encouraged to be active and who have plenty of opportunities to play with family and friends, develop good coordination skills. This in turn increases their enjoyment of physical activities.

Toddlers and young children like seeing everyone around them, especially brothers and sisters, being active and having fun. Young children learn by watching others and having active role models increases children's self-efficacy, which means their confidence to perform a skill.

Family activities are ideal. They improve everybody's health and help children to learn that being active is fun, no matter what your age or size. As parents and activity role models we can teach our children simple outdoor games that all children love to play, so that they can join in with friends and at playgroups.

Take it easy

If your children haven't been particularly active up till now, start off gradually. It's tough for children to go from relatively little activity to a full-on action-packed day. Small steps build up a child's self-confidence and enjoyment and are the best way to create a lasting active lifestyle.

Just spending more time outdoors automatically increases physical activity. Young children enjoy helping their parents with grown-up tasks, so make the most of this (before they start demanding pocket money without lifting a finger) and get them to help you wash the car, rake up

JUST CHANGE ONE THING

Be positive about your child's efforts. Praise and encouragement can make all the difference to a child's confidence and commitment to a sport or activity. Support and encouragement build self-esteem and motivation. Criticism is downright discouraging.

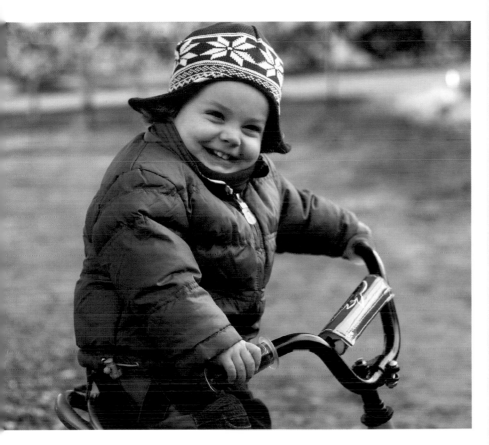

Join in with the children

Jen was keen to be a good activity role model for her children and signed up for a keep-fit class to show them how committed she was to being active. The trouble was, she didn't really want to go – it was making her feel miserable and she wasn't very good at hiding the fact.

Being active doesn't have to mean doing structured exercise and sports. There are lots of ways to be active round the home or actually joining in with the children, especially if they are still quite young. Once Jen realised she could get just as much exercise – and have lots more fun – simply chasing the children round the garden and squirting them with the hose, she cancelled her keep-fit class and never looked back. The children love it when she joins in and have persuaded her to buy them all a trampoline.

leaves, sweep paths or help with more specialised garden jobs like planting seeds or weeding – but be prepared for a few mishaps.

Going outside loses its appeal in winter but often the thought is worse than the reality. Children aren't bothered about the cold and, wrapped up warmly, still enjoy playing outside or going for a walk.

Ideal garden toys (if you have space) include trikes, bikes, scooters, roller skates. If you're on a budget, look in charity shops, where you can often find toys in good condition. Another idea is to join your local Freecycle website and see what you can pick up online (www.freecycle.org.uk).

Set a good example

It's no good sending the children out to play and then just sitting around indoors yourself. You've got to be a good role model. If you sign your children up for a sports club, you need to do the same for yourself. An inactive parent sends the message that while it's important to be active as a child, it's ok to be sluggish as an adult.

Adding-on exercise

Nicky has two young daughters, Becky and Jess. She wanted them to be more active but after a long day at work she didn't have the energy to go out and play with them.

You don't have to treat activity as separate from everyday life. If there clearly isn't room to add new activities without making you feel stressed out, you need to think laterally and see what you can add-on to things you already do. So instead of driving to the duck pond to feed the ducks, Nicky realised she and the girls could walk instead. And on Sundays they walk nearly a mile to grandad's house for tea – and he drives them home afterwards. Just look for small ways to boost the activities you already do and you'll notice the difference.

Being an activity provider for toddlers and young children

Toddlers and young children are constantly on the move. In fact they're likely to keep you on the go all day too. So all you really need to do is guide them in the right direction from time to time. Their interests and skills are constantly developing so you need to keep challenging them with new and different activities.

Get outside

Young children love spending time outside and research shows that children who play outside tend to be more active overall. The other benefit of being outside is that the tv and computer are out of sight and out of mind.

It might come as a bit of a surprise but children prefer being active to sitting around. When

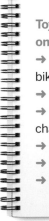
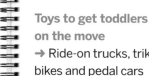

Toys to get toddlers on the move
→ Ride-on trucks, trikes, bikes and pedal cars
→ Pull-along animals
→ Dolls' pram or dolls' push chair – for boys and girls
→ Climbing frame
→ Slide
→ Swings

young children do watch tv or play computer games, it's often only because they're bored and can't think of what to do. Give them a few ideas and they'll be off outside like a shot. Research has shown that they prefer to play, so take advantage of it – you're pushing at an open door.

Everyday physical activity isn't just about playing or sports. An easy way to get children to be active is to make movement as natural to them as breathing. Good ways to do this include encouraging children to walk everywhere – to preschool, to school, to the shops, to the playground, to visit friends. Get rid of the pushchair as soon as you can – or keep it in the garage for emergencies only.

Building up confidence

Early childhood is the ideal time to build a child's self esteem about being active. Research shows that parents who have confidence in their children's ability actually help increase the children's motivation. Having said that, most young children arc too young to enjoy competitive sports. They'll have much more fun doing things where they can measure their own progress, such as swimming and ice skating.

Make sure everyone in the family

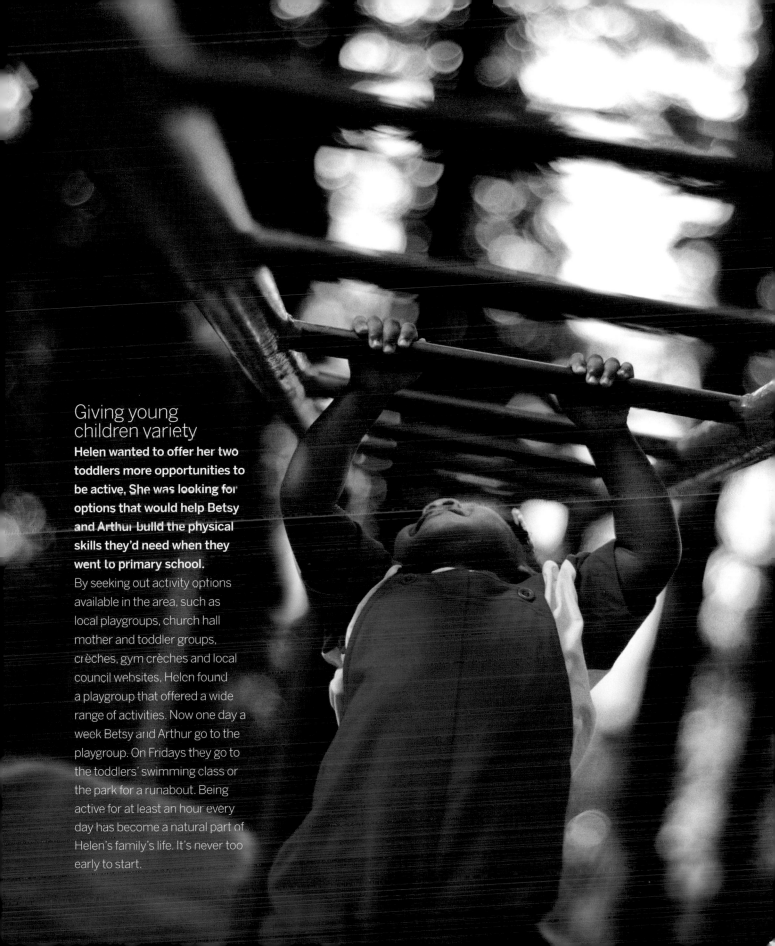

Giving young children variety

Helen wanted to offer her two toddlers more opportunities to be active. She was looking for options that would help Betsy and Arthur build the physical skills they'd need when they went to primary school.

By seeking out activity options available in the area, such as local playgroups, church hall mother and toddler groups, crèches, gym crèches and local council websites, Helen found a playgroup that offered a wide range of activities. Now one day a week Betsy and Arthur go to the playgroup. On Fridays they go to the toddlers' swimming class or the park for a runabout. Being active for at least an hour every day has become a natural part of Helen's family's life. It's never too early to start.

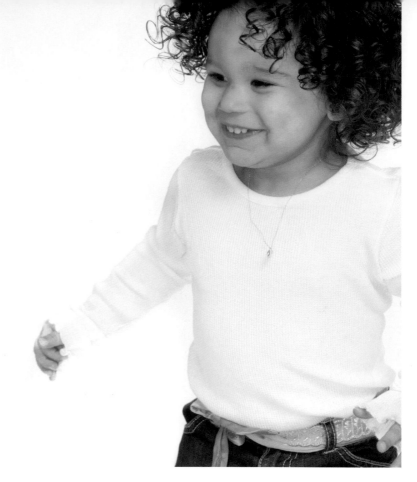

Rainy day activities

Jemma wasn't sure how to make sure her small children got enough activity on days when it was too wet to go outside.

Young children love dancing. It's easy enough to make a cd of favourite family songs that will get them singing and dancing along for half an hour.

gets equal treatment. Focusing on a child who is naturally athletic and neglecting to encourage less able siblings may be a natural reaction but less athletic brothers and sisters can easily become discouraged. One study showed that parents tended to give more encouragement to their sons, with the result that the daughters felt less capable and were less enthusiastic. Try not to fall into the same trap.

Being an activity enforcer for toddlers and young children

Toddlers and young children need boundaries and creating a daily routine that includes lots of playtime and a little bit of children's tv or a video will give them a sense of security and familiarity. Your job as an activity enforcer tends to be easier when the children are younger as they are more likely to go along with the rules – especially when they are consistent.

Many parents have found that having a set routine – almost like a timetable – works well. Setting a specific time for active play, whether it's after breakfast, after an afternoon sleep or before lunch – is a good idea. Similarly, having a set time for watching tv or a video also helps. In winter you will have to spend more time indoors but there are still lots of ways to keep toddlers on the move, such as an indoor treasure hunt; an obstacle course of old boxes, blankets and chairs; hide-and-seek; or good old-fashioned hunt the thimble.

Don't put a tv in your toddler's bedroom. Research has shown that preschool children who have a tv in their bedroom are more likely to gain excess weight. It's much easier to enforce limits on watching tv and videos if the tv is downstairs in the sitting room.

Support your children in any way you can, by inviting friends to play and by buying them outdoor play equipment. Look for activity centres in your area: indoor soft-play children's areas with ladders, slides and the popular 'ball pools' are pretty much standard all over the country and a great place to meet up with friends. (Visit www.softplayareas.co.uk)

Don't bribe children to be active. Promising a reward or a treat for being active gives the message that activity is a job that requires payment. The reward – which is often a food treat – becomes more important than the activity.

Always ask

If you're planning to take your child to pre-school or nursery school, find out in advance what sort of activities they have on offer. Is there an outdoor play area? And what play equipment do they have? What sort of indoor activities do the children do?

If your child spends time with a childminder, tell them what you would like your child to do. Be clear and concise: communication is all important when it comes to setting guidelines.

Activity isn't enough on its own

Pauline's toddlers were on the go all the time so she was confident that they were getting enough exercise and she felt justified in letting them watch tv when they felt like it. She also tended to put on the tv when she was too busy to spend time with them.

A healthy-weight home encourages increased physical activity as well as reducing the amount of time the family spends watching tv. Although Pauline's family is fine at the moment, too much time in front of the tv can lead to weight gain. Once she understood this, she started to pay more attention to how much tv the children were watching.

Great games for young children

- **Hide-and-seek** – indoors and out. Just make sure you set a few rules, such as no hiding in mum's wardrobe, don't trample the flower beds
- **Ball games** like Piggy in the Middle
- **It** – make sure you're on hand to intervene and see that everyone gets a go at being 'it'
- **What's the Time, Mr Wolf?** Everyone runs around until the wolf says it's dinnertime, then they make a dash for 'home' – a tree, wall, garden bench, etc
- **Skipping** – either individually or get a long piece of washing line from the ironmongers, tie one end to the fence and get everyone jumping in together
- **Hopscotch** – draw squares with chalk on the patio or drive, or play on the pavement if you live in a quiet street

Set a good example

Ann was concerned at the amount of time her son Toby spent on his computer and playing video games. She admitted that she also spent a lot of time online each day.

If you want your children to cut down on screen time then you've got to look at your own behaviour and become an activity role model. Ann decided to make a big effort to cut back on the time she spent online and try to spend more time outside – walking the dog, gardening and going for bike rides. She encouraged Toby to join her when he took screen breaks. He was reluctant at first but when he did get out for a bit he met up with other boys in the neighbourhood, who started asking him to play football or to go off on their bikes. In the end he got the balance right and enjoyed playing outside with friends, which helped him to stick to Rules 3 and 4 – being active for at least an hour a day and limiting screen time to two hours a day.

older children

Being an activity role model for older children

As parents, we can still be activity role models for older children. They don't miss a trick and will be very aware of whether or not we take part in family activities or have our own sport or class that we take part in. By joining a squash club or taking up yoga and by going on family bike rides or walks, we're demonstrating the importance of being active, as well as showing that we think it's fun and enjoyable.

Research clearly shows that children with active parents tend to be more active, while children whose parents have a more sedentary lifestyle tend to be less active.

Older children tend to have quite a busy schedule, with school, homework and friends taking up a lot of time. Most secondary school timetables have around two hours a week of PE so days can go by without them being active. But if you're active yourself you can show your children that it is possible to fit in activity as part of a busy lifestyle. Get them being active as part of daily routine and it's likely to be a habit that sticks. Easy ways to get them on the move include, where practical, walking to school or cycling, if it's safe; or joining a lunchtime or after-school sports club. In summer it's easy to send the children out on their bikes after school, or to play football at the park or to take the dog for a walk.

In winter you need to be more imaginative – if you have space in the living room, lots of children like bouncing around on big indoor exercise balls. Even on chilly days the lure of the garden trampoline can be irresistible – provided it isn't raining – and they won't feel cold once they get moving. Similarly, winter bike rides or brisk walks can be invigorating and just the thing to snap children out of their couch-potato lethargy.

Let them choose a class at your local leisure centre: there are all sorts of options, everything from martial arts like judo or taekwondo to dance classes like jazz or salsa. Swimming is a great all-year-round option and a good family activity. Many pools have challenging flumes or giant inflatables to tempt children to stay active for longer.

At half term or in the holidays, get the children to think of places they can go for a day out. Put a chart on the wall and use pictures from

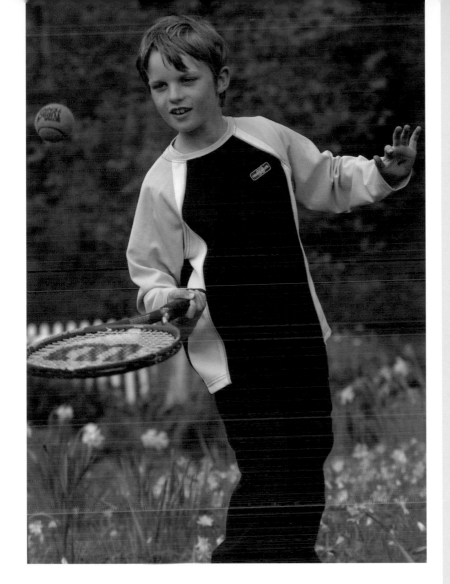

Celia realised the whole family was watching far too much tv and she wanted everyone to cut down. But her son Max was a keen sportsman and led a very active lifestyle and liked to relax by watching tv at the end of the day. She was worried that he might feel resentful at having to stick to the rules when he already followed a healthy-weight lifestyle.

It can be tough to start clamping down on behaviour when one member of the family already seems to be getting things right. But for the 5 Simple Rules to work they have to be followed consistently and they have to apply to all family members, not just those with a weight problem. In the end Celia was surprised at how easy it was to reduce the family's screen time and she was pleased that Max soon found other ways to relax like listening to music and reading sports magazines.

a theme park brochure or sports centre to illustrate it. Wherever you go, make sure that you walk, cycle or run at least part of the way.

Being an activity provider for older children

Older children have quite different reasons for being active – it's less about having fun and much more about being competitive. Ask any school child and they will be able to tell you who is the fastest in the class, who is the best at football, who's the strongest. By keeping this in mind you'll be able to find an activity or sport to engage your child. Peer pressure will also motivate your child but you still have a vital role to play – it will just be different, like giving them a lift to matches, buying equipment and kit and generally being enthusiastic.

The Olympics are coming so there will be more talk about sports. Is there one activity, such as archery or swimming, that you can get your children interested in?

Start with the line of least resistance

Ginny came up with the idea of shortening three of the 5 Simple Rules to the expression 5-2-1. That's five daily portions of fruit and vegetables, no more than two hours of screen time and at least one hour of activity. But she ran into trouble with her husband Alan's resistance to the screen time rule.

When a family is struggling with one of the rules it often helps to focus on the changes they are willing to make and put the difficult rule on the back burner for a while. Ginny decided to be positive and concentrate on being active. She encouraged Alan to take the children to the park to play football and planned active weekends featuring bike rides, family walks on the beach and following forest trails. She reckoned that, with time, the extra activity should start to overcome Alan's resistance to cutting down on tv.

Positive feedback

Older children thrive on positive feedback and encouragement, whether from their parents, brothers and sisters or friends – research has shown that it motivates them to be more active. Children in general and girls in particular are more active when they know they've got their parents' backing.

Use an older child's competitive streak to motivate them. As well as competing against their friends, they can also break their own records by setting themselves personal goals in sports like running or at the gym – on the rowing machine or cross-trainer.

As with younger children, being active means less time for sitting around watching tv or playing computer games. Older children have even more distractions – watching their favourite soaps, texting, online chat rooms, computer games, not to mention the time they actually need to be at the computer researching their homework. Typically, older children spend five hours 20 minutes a day watching tv or sitting in front of a computer – five years ago it was four hours and 40 minutes. We need to bring this right down in the healthy-weight home.

Being an activity enforcer for older children

This is when the role of enforcer gets tough. Rejecting authority is part of growing up – as is challenging adults. The trick is to find a way of motivating older children – and limiting screen time – without ending up with an all-out rebellion on your hands.

Older children will need different types of support, such as buying sports equipment. As parents we can help by making sure our

---

Typical teenage excuses – and how to answer them back

● **None of my friends do it** – Be the first and who knows, you might start a craze

● **I don't like team sports** – Then try something solitary like rock climbing, quad biking or archery

● **I don't want to get hot and sweaty** – Everyone else will be doing the same so no one's likely to notice

● **Sport isn't cool** – What would Cristiano Ronaldo or Kelly Holmes have to say about that?

● **I'm embarrassed about wearing shorts** – Ask your PE teacher/ instructor if you can wear tracksuit bottoms instead

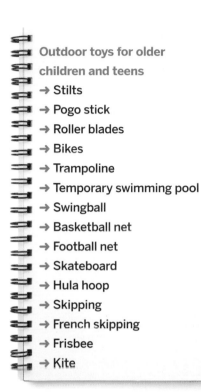

Outdoor toys for older children and teens
→ Stilts
→ Pogo stick
→ Roller blades
→ Bikes
→ Trampoline
→ Temporary swimming pool
→ Swingball
→ Basketball net
→ Football net
→ Skateboard
→ Hula hoop
→ Skipping
→ French skipping
→ Frisbee
→ Kite

children have the right gear – clothing that fits, the right footwear, and all the equipment they need. Praise, showing an interest and going to matches or events are all powerful ways to motivate older children and to show them that you have confidence in their ability.

This is the phase when many teenagers will probably want to drop out of family activities and do things on their own. Letting them choose their own thing – such as dance, martial arts, trampolining, fencing, horse riding – means they are more likely to stick to their choice.

Arrange an outing or give them tickets for a birthday treat to a musical to inspire them. Matinees are often cheaper and if you book ahead you're more likely to get a bargain. National Express, Stagecoach and other transport companies have excursions to shows all over the UK at competitive prices.

Setting goals can help motivate older children. Many activities have levels to work towards – certificates for distance in swimming for example, belt levels in judo. Discuss with your child what is a reasonable goal and help them to get there. It's a great confidence booster.

You can also set goals to help teens reduce the time they spend in front of the tv or computer.

Be a role model too

For older children you've got to be a role model as well as an enforcer or they won't take you seriously. The familiar saying, 'Do as I say, not as I do' just won't cut any ice with them. Research shows that older children and teenagers are more likely to take part in after-school activities when both parents are active too. In contrast, children whose parents watched more than two hours of tv a day tended to be more sedentary. Remember, Rules 3 and 4 apply to everyone in the family.

Going it alone

Jill's 12-year-old son Stuart was keen to be more active but didn't want to do team sports and felt he wasn't yet in good enough shape to use the gym at the local sports centre.

There are plenty of options for boys and girls who prefer solo exercise. Jill found out that her local fitness centre offered individual sessions with a personal trainer to show Stuart exercises that he could then carry on and do at home. To improve his general fitness levels and stamina, Jill also organised some family activities like bike rides and country walks.

looking after your children

One of a parent's most important jobs is making sure that their children are safe, which involves taking on the role of protector. Being a protector can mean anything from defending a child who is being bullied to standing up for a child's right to fair treatment from their teachers.

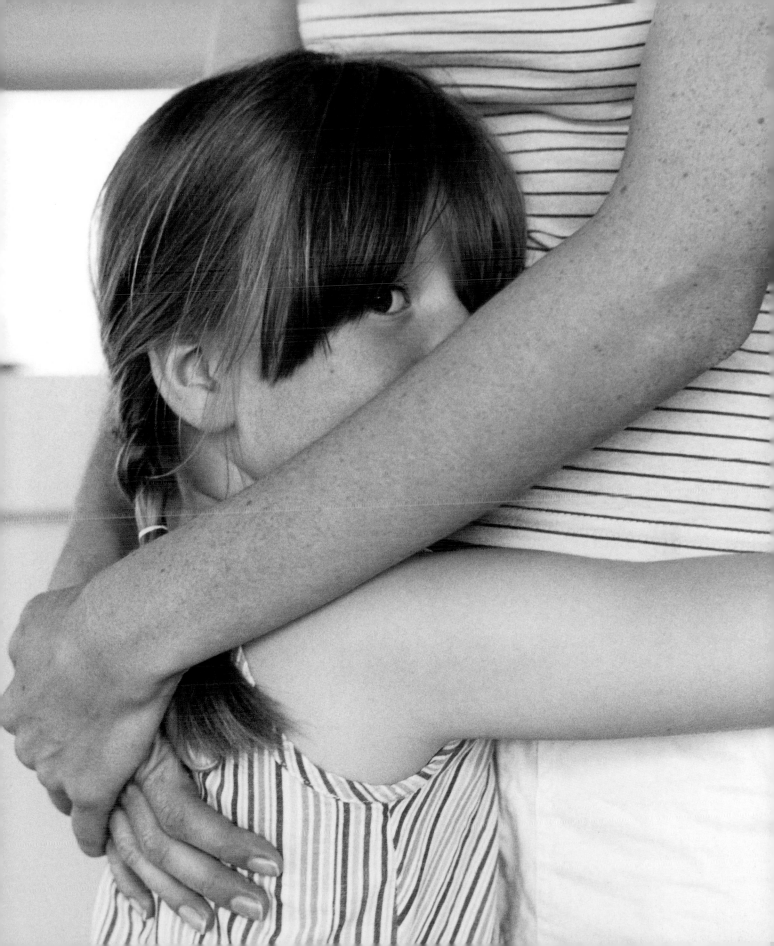

Kitchen clear-out

Ron and Maria wanted to rethink the contents of their kitchen cupboards to make it easier for them to lose weight and to help one of their daughters achieve a healthy weight too – their younger daughter didn't have a weight problem.

Creating a healthy-weight home has to involve all members of the family. Ron agreed to stop bringing home sweets and chocolates after work while Maria stopped drinking soft drinks and had water with meals instead and herb teas in between. The fridge was stocked with healthy snacks like carrot and celery sticks and low-fat dips, and there was always fruit on the table. And everyone in the family ate the same foods.

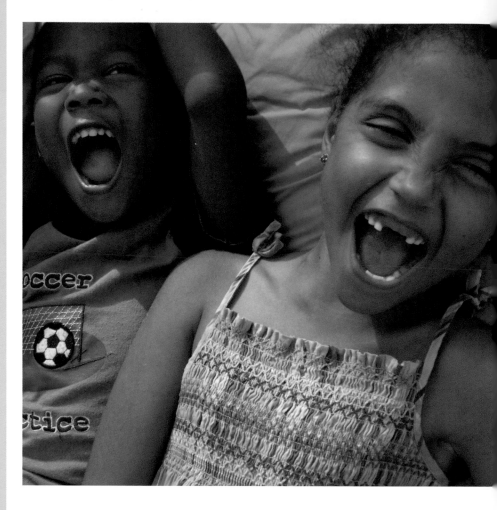

Protection and guidance

As parents, we create the family structure in which our children grow and develop. But children also learn about the social relationships that are part of everyday life by meeting up with friends and neighbours, going to school, to clubs or to church. The relationships our children develop in the community can form a strong support system as they grow older and have to deal with everything that life throws at them.

One of our first jobs as protector, if we have more than one child, is to manage the relationships between siblings. These important bonds can affect our ability to maintain a healthy-weight home. It's quite common for children to deal with unresolved sibling conflict by rebelling against the 5 Simple Rules, and you, as the protector, will have to decide how deeply to get involved in your children's

> **An effective healthy-weight protector**
> → guides children when they deal with conflict
> → helps them make difficult decisions
> → encourages activities
> → supports children who have weight issues

arguments. Research can help you come to a decision: one study showed that it is helpful for parents to intervene and keep the peace between young children; but when children get older, interfering parents can actually make things worse.

The role of protector also draws on other roles – provider, enforcer and role model – to keep our children safe. Feeling protected by an adult is an essential element in helping children to find their way in the world.

Children are more likely to be successful when they are guided and encouraged to take part in family, school and community activities. Parents need to steer children in the right direction and help them make sensible decisions. But as our children grow up, we have to step back and gradually let go of the role of protector, letting our children take more and more responsibility for their decisions and actions – including those related to the 5 Simple Rules.

What does a healthy-weight protector do?

While all children need protection, those with weight issues can be in greater need. It can be hard to find the right level of protection – too much or too little can both create problems. What we do know is that it is vital to treat all children in the family in the same way when creating a healthy-weight home. Singling out an overweight child for special treatment doesn't help anyone.

Protecting an overweight child from prejudice is one of the toughest jobs any parent faces. The sad reality is that children tend to react less favourably to heavy children than those in the normal weight range. In one study, children responded more negatively to drawings of heavy children today than a similar study group back in the early 1960s – which suggests the stigma of excess weight in children is greater today than it was nearly 50 years ago. The bias against excess weight can begin as early as preschool, where it's been shown that children prefer to play with thin or average-weight

Dealing with peer pressure

Chris was 16 and battling with his weight. He had really taken on board the 5 Simple Rules, especially Rule 1 – focus on wholesome nutritious foods – and he had started to notice the difference in the way he felt. But he told Scott, his dad, that his friends had started to tease him when they were out, making fun of his healthy choices from the menu in the local café and trying to tempt him with chips and burgers. He asked Scott what he should do about it.

Friends can be downright unhelpful when you're really making an effort to turn your life around. From talking with Chris, Scott discovered that he was proud of his achievements so far and that his new eating habits were making him healthier. Scott praised his commitment and reminded him to keep his long-term goal in mind at all times. He pointed out to Chris that just because his friends were skinnier than him didn't mean that they were any healthier. With his confidence boosted, Chris felt better able to deal with his friends' comments.

When only one child is overweight

Matt and Micha wanted to help their teenage daughter Jessica who has a weight problem. They have two more teenagers, Chloe and Jude, both of whom are within the normal weight range for their ages. Matt and Micha felt that if they all followed the 5 Simple Rules, they'd all be making sacrifices for the sake of one family member.

To create a healthy-weight home everyone in the family has to follow the 5 Simple Rules. It doesn't help to see them as some kind of sacrifice or penance. Matt and Micha needed to focus on the health benefits that all the family will gain – from having more energy to feeling fitter and having a general sense of well-being. They knew they'd have to keep an eye on each other to make sure that they were treating all three children fairly and not being extra strict with Jessica or too lenient with Chloe and Jude. As well as sticking consistently to the 5 Simple Rules, they decided to make all mention of weight, weight loss, body fat and things like clothes sizes strictly off limits. This made it easier to put a lid on name-calling and bickering and arguing about following the rules.

children. Chapter 13 has useful information on getting advice from professionals for parents who need help in dealing with these sorts of situations. Bullying is a real threat that should not be ignored. Bullies often pick on overweight children, and adults must intervene and protect their child. Many parents get help from support groups, telephone helplines, by reading

OVERWEIGHT CHILDREN CAN HAVE A LOWER SELF-IMAGE AND SENSE OF WORTH COMPARED TO OTHER CHILDREN

up on the topic and sometimes by seeking professional help such as counselling to help a child cope.

Minimising conflict

In a healthy-weight home young children can need protecting from situations that put them into conflict with the 5 Simple Rules. For example, a grandparent who thinks that treats are a reward for good behaviour or a friend who openly makes comments about a child's weight: in situations like these, a parent must step in on behalf of the child, to limit how often they occur and to find new strategies to help them stick to the 5 Simple Rules.

Boosting self-esteem

In a healthy-weight home the protector needs to boost and maintain the self-esteem of a child with weight issues. Overweight children can have a lower self-image and sense of worth compared to children with a healthy body weight. Self-esteem tends to dip anyway when children enter their teens, no matter what they weigh. It's something to keep an eye on because low self-esteem is linked to feelings of sadness, loneliness and nervousness, along with an increased tendency to smoke or drink. Children with low self-esteem can also develop behaviour problems. They can become trapped in a vicious circle when their negative feelings reduce their motivation to follow the 5 Simple Rules. If this seems to be happening to your child it's important to recognise and praise even the smallest efforts your child is making.

Helping your child choose the right activity

In our role as protector we can have a big impact on the level of physical activity that our children achieve over time. Research shows that an active childhood often leads to continued regular physical activity during teen years and on into adulthood. Lifelong physical

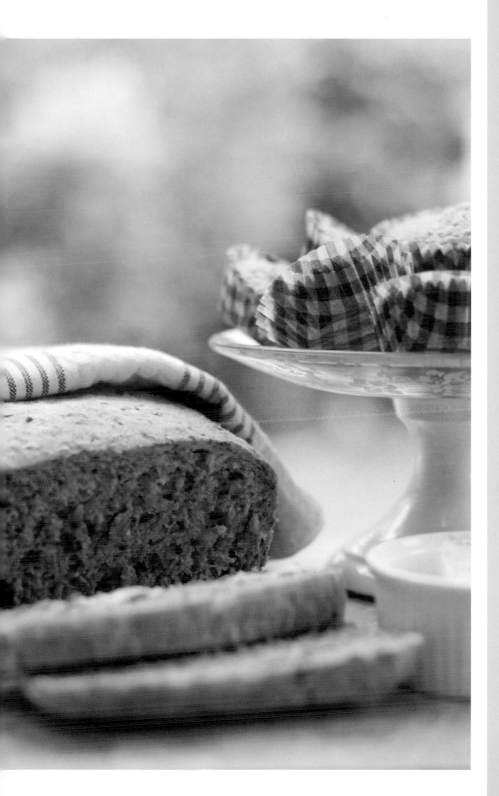

Diabetes in the family

Tina was worried because diabetes runs in the family. Her husband Patrick has type 2 diabetes and her eldest daughter Jade has the same build as her dad. Tina was very aware that she didn't want to single out Jade for special treatment.

While heavier children may be more at risk of developing diabetes, creating a healthy-weight home will help protect everyone in the family. Instead of telling everyone that she was changing their lifestyle to help with Jade's weight, Tina said that she wanted all of them to be healthier and she also wanted to take special care of dad. She switched to wholegrain bread and low-fat spread, and put more fruit and veg on the table. The strategy worked: Jade lost weight without even trying and everyone felt fit and healthy.

Tackling bullies

12-year-old Alex was being picked on and bullied on the school bus because of his weight. His parents Jane and Andrew wanted to find the best way to help him deal with the situation.

To boost Alex's self-esteem and confidence, Andrew started spending more time with Alex, taking him bowling, going for long walks and working together on the car. This also gave him the chance to check how Alex was feeling and how he was doing in other areas at school. Jane contacted the school to let them know what was going on and they suggested Alex join the school mentoring scheme, teaming him up with an older boy who'd had a similar experience when he was younger so knew exactly how he was feeling. The school also contacted the bus company to ask them to keep an eye on what was going on.

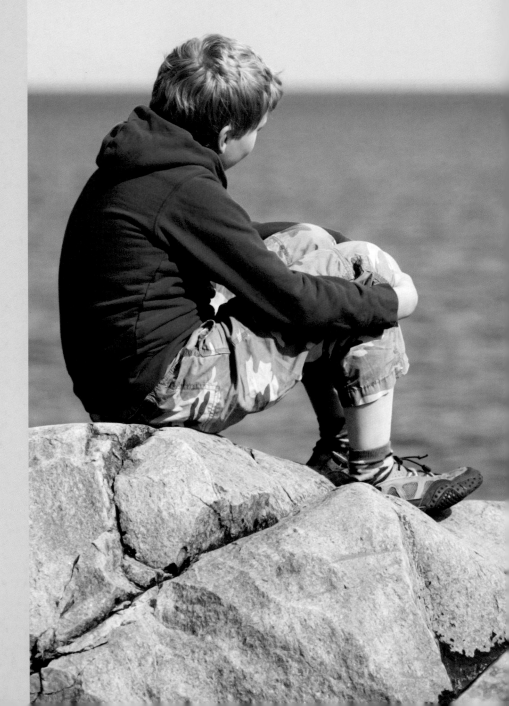

PROTECTORS HELP CHILDREN CHOOSE ACTIVITIES THAT ARE APPROPRIATE FOR THEIR AGE AND WEIGHT

activity has not only health and weight benefits but emotional ones too – that well-known feel-good factor you get after a good work out or a cross-country run.

Protectors help children choose activities that are appropriate for their age and weight. Overweight children are physically different from children at a healthy weight and are less able to tackle energetic exercise and sports. Because their bodies are larger and heavier, they have to work harder to do the same activity as a lighter child, which means they'll also tire more quickly. Overweight children are also more prone to sprains and other sports-type injuries. Forcing an overweight child to exercise beyond their capabilities to speed up weight loss is likely to backfire – firstly, because they won't enjoy it, and secondly, because it may even cause injury.

Activity and socialising

Lots of activities can be quite sociable and involve chatting with friends when you meet up for your weekly yoga class, challenging friends to a squash match, meeting new people when you swap partners at a salsa class. Teenage girls in particular can find this kind of social contact excruciating, and worry about negative comments from their peers about their body weight or shape. They may be embarrassed to exercise with friends or hate getting undressed in communal changing rooms or feel uncomfortable in shorts or a swimsuit.

In one study, girls said that one of the main reasons that they were not physically active was that they were self-conscious about their appearance. With any luck it will be a passing phase, but if it's happening to your daughter you still need to do something about it. Approach her school to find out whether there's a school counsellor or mentor who can offer support or who can organise a support group for girls with weight issues, to help them handle the social aspects. Support groups help by letting children know they're not alone, lessening their concerns and boosting self-esteem.

At home encourage your daughter to keep active in other ways such as walking the dog, going for a bike ride or exercising at home to a dvd. If she is still happy to join in with family activities,

Non-competitive fun

Gwen and Jim were stumped. They couldn't come up with an activity that appealed to their daughter Ellie, who made it plain she didn't want to compete in team sports. Horse riding is a great way for girls to get active and get lots of fresh air. Ellie found that she liked being in control of such a powerful animal and developed a bond with her favourite horse. As she got fitter she also helped out with mucking out in return for an extra half hour's ride every now and then.

Make things clear

Leanne was frustrated with Phillip her ex-husband. When their daughter Rebecca spent a weekend with him he took her food shopping and when she chose a readymade pizza that wasn't particularly nutritious or wholesome, he stocked up by buying several more for the freezer.

As a protector it is Leanne's job to make sure that everyone looking after Rebecca understands the principles of a healthy-weight home – and that includes Phillip. By sitting down and explaining the 5 Simple Rules, especially Rule 1 (focus on wholesome nutritious meals), she helped him understand that healthy food was a priority at home and should be so at his home too. If the pizza was going to be a treat for the day, that was fine, but buying several at once sends the message that it's an everyday food rather than a treat. To help Phillip and Rebecca make healthy choices when they are out shopping she told Phillip about the Traffic Light code on packaging and explained that he could stock up on mainly 'green' foods but to go easy on amber and red (see page 96 for more details).

these are often less fraught than exercising with a group of friends. Family bike rides can boost confidence and self-esteem, as well as increasing stamina and physical fitness.

Focus on the strong points

In one study, children who were overweight were assessed in various areas of ability: while they had average scores for academic ability, behaviour and even athletic ability, they scored much lower than their healthy-weight contemporaries in terms of self-worth, physical appearance and

FOCUSING ON A CHILD'S STRENGTHS AND BUILDING UP THEIR CONFIDENCE IN WEAKER AREAS CAN MAKE A DIFFERENCE

peer acceptance. Focusing on a child's strengths and building up their confidence in weaker areas can make a real difference – and so does recognising and praising their efforts to get down to a healthy weight.

Expressing confidence in a child's physical ability also helps. Research shows that children whose parents express confidence in them feel supported and feel motivated to carry on. When

children themselves become confident in their physical abilities, they're much more likely to want to join in with sports and activities. Not surprisingly, it also helps if they enjoy the activity – it's a factor that's closely linked with them wanting to join in.

Don't make excuses

It might seem like a brainwave to protect your child by explaining away their weight problem as a medical issue. However, research has shown that although younger children may be more accepting of a heavy child with health problems, older children are far less sympathetic in general and react negatively.

Beware well-meaning friends

Whether knowingly or otherwise, friends – and even members of the family – can sabotage the best efforts to create a healthy-weight home. While parents enforce the 5 Simple Rules within the family, they may also need to shield children from others who are not so supportive. Protectors are duty bound to spread the word about the 5 Simple Rules to childminders, extended family and regular visitors. One area that often needs to be explained to others is the family's policy against using treats as a reward.

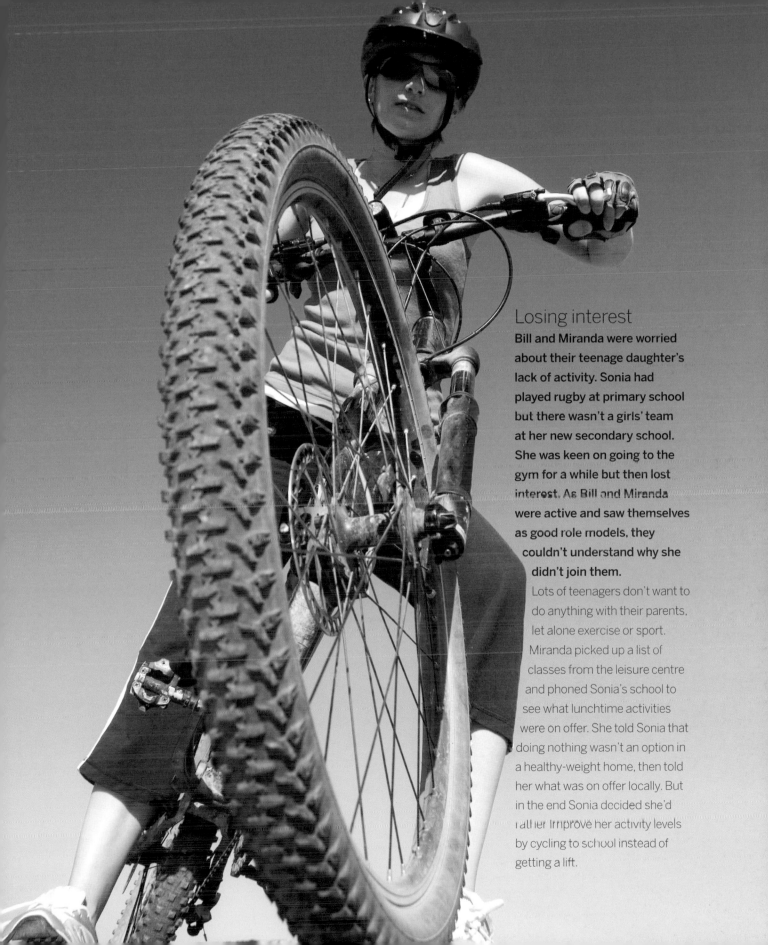

Losing interest

Bill and Miranda were worried about their teenage daughter's lack of activity. Sonia had played rugby at primary school but there wasn't a girls' team at her new secondary school. She was keen on going to the gym for a while but then lost interest. As Bill and Miranda were active and saw themselves as good role models, they couldn't understand why she didn't join them.

Lots of teenagers don't want to do anything with their parents, let alone exercise or sport. Miranda picked up a list of classes from the leisure centre and phoned Sonia's school to see what lunchtime activities were on offer. She told Sonia that doing nothing wasn't an option in a healthy-weight home, then told her what was on offer locally. But in the end Sonia decided she'd rather improve her activity levels by cycling to school instead of getting a lift.

taking the message outside the home

Once you've made positive changes at home, you'll want to spread the word beyond your front door. This is the time to think about becoming an agent for change and taking the healthy-weight message out into your local community.

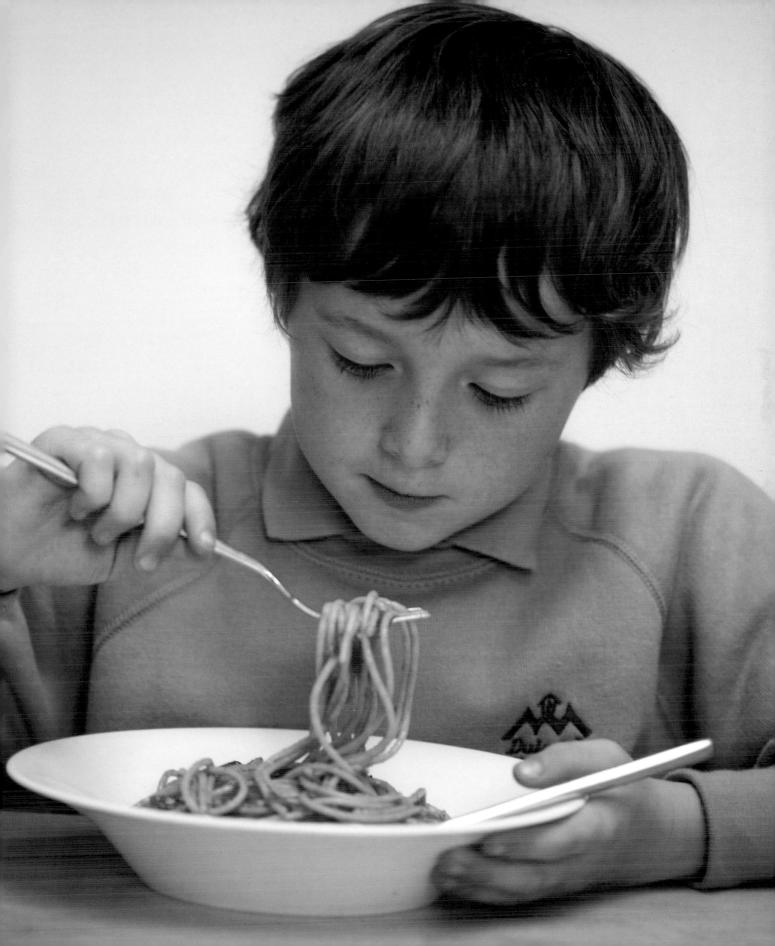

Take it slowly

Jo's daughter Millie is at secondary school and the caterers decided to re-stock the canteen well in advance of government guidelines. Overnight the fizzy drinks disappeared, along with doughnuts and muffins and chips. In came low-fat yoghurts, salads, wholemeal sandwiches, wraps and baked potatoes. Jo overheard Millie and her friends moaning that there was nothing for them to eat any more.

With hindsight it would have been better for the caterers to have made the changes slowly, cutting back on chips and bringing in jacket potatoes gradually, phasing out fizzy drinks slowly – just giving the students time to get used to change and time to try out new foods before switching over completely. The caterers are hoping to tempt students back into the canteen by planning theme days and taster days with free samples.

Agents for change

To stand any chance of reversing the trend in childhood obesity, we need to make changes in two different areas: our day-to-day environment – our homes, schools and communities; and the wider environment, covering everything from food production and supply, to how food is advertised and how nutrition is taught in schools.

Agents for change tend to be most effective when they focus on a specific issue and work at the level with which they are most comfortable – and, being realistic, for most of us parents that's going to be locally. One good way to get started is to network with other parents to see how they feel and what they are doing or are prepared to do to change things they feel strongly about.

Start with schools

Our children spend nearly as much time at school as they do at home so it makes sense for them to follow healthy-weight guidelines there too. An obvious starting point is the food that schools serve. There's been a huge shake up in school canteens across the country. New government standards are already in place in primary schools and while secondary schools have slightly longer to implement the changes,

many are already following the new guidelines in advance of the deadline, when it will be against the law for canteens to sell or serve sweets, chocolate, fizzy drinks and crisps. While cakes and biscuits aren't banned, they can only be served as part of a full meal at lunchtime, and chips and other fried foods are only on the menu for a maximum of twice a week. Positive changes include serving oily fish at least every three weeks, plenty of fruit and veg every day, bread to fill up on and drinking water that's free and easily available – no more thirsty children sticking their heads under the tap in the cloakroom. You'll find full details on what schools should be serving in a booklet for parents called *School Food: Changing for the Better* by The School Food

NETWORK WITH OTHER PARENTS TO SEE HOW THEY FEEL AND WHAT THEY ARE PREPARED TO DO

Trust. Download a copy at www.schoolfoodtrust.org.uk/index.asp; click on 'Parents and carers' and then on 'booklet' in the text.

The government has invested millions in making sure that children get a healthy meal at lunchtime but the success of the scheme still depends on parents being involved every step of the way. If we don't back our schools, a lot of good work can be undone.

Taking it further

Schools should now be serving less processed food and more freshly cooked food, meals should be healthier and more balanced, and students should have better choices at lunchtime. But if you feel your school still isn't getting it right, there are things you can do as an agent for change.

● Put pressure on the Local Education Authority and the catering company it uses, to improve the quality of the food on offer. To help you work out who to contact, download the leaflet from Jamie Oliver's *School Dinners* website: www.channel4.com/life/microsites/J/jamies_school_dinners. Click on 'Do Something' then 'Make a Difference'.

● If putting pressure on doesn't work, suggest the school tries a new catering firm.

● Create your own school meals company. If you're really committed this can be a rewarding way to change things, but it's not for the faint-hearted. You'll need a business plan to put in a tender to supply school meals. The backing of other parents, governors, teachers (and pupils) is essential.

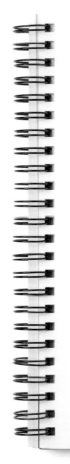

How to back up your school

● Have faith in the catering company and encourage your child to have school dinners. They are far more likely to try new foods when friends – and teachers – are doing the same.

● Ask if parents can have lunch in the canteen from time to time. That way you can keep an eye on whether the school caterers are sticking to government standards. If you have any worries, talk to the head teacher or caterer to work out how to put things right. Equally, if you think they're doing a great job, say so.

● Don't undermine school standards. If your child wants to take a packed lunch rather than buy lunch in the canteen, send them to school with food and drink that matches the standards – that means no crisps, chocolate or fizzy drinks.

● If you give your children money to spend on the way to school – or on the way home – encourage them to buy healthier snacks rather than fizzy drinks, crisps, chocolate and chewing gum, which are now banned in schools.

One determined mum in Kent was the starting point for a catering company that now provides freshly cooked meals to 21 schools using local produce (see page 136). The Soil Association has produced a very useful action pack called *Food For Life* to help interested parents improve the school catering system or help set up their own in-school catering company. Go to www.foodforlife.org.uk/resources/action and download the School Meals Action Pack.

parent power works

Stephanie Hayman, parent governor at Warden House Primary School in Deal in Kent and mum of Harry in Year 5, had been worried for some time about the quality of food served at school. 'I felt we weren't getting it right and it's such an important aspect of the school day.'

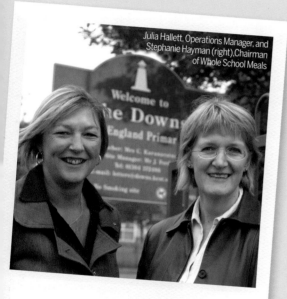

Julia Hallett, Operations Manager, and Stephanie Hayman (right), Chairman of Whole School Meals

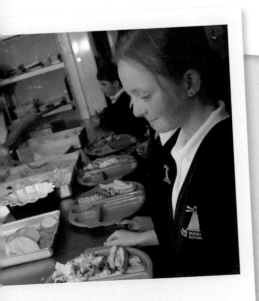

When Stephanie heard that the Local Education Authority was putting out the school meals contract to tender in 2006, she knew it was now or never if she was going to do something about school food. So she talked to other governors, parents and teachers to see how they felt about setting up their own catering company, to bring control over meals back where it belonged – in school. Her vision was to serve freshly cooked meals prepared from scratch using local produce.

What really helped her decision to go ahead was Kent County Council's plan to break down catering contracts into regional areas, so she called a meeting of the heads of the 21 schools in their 'cluster' to test the water. And they said: 'Go for it'.

A local newspaper published an article about her plan, attracting plenty of attention. From the people who came forward to help,

she formed a core of directors, including a restaurant owner, a very experienced school governor and a retired director from a cross-channel ferry company. And so Whole School Meals was formed.

The first thing they did was to draw up a constitution and create a limited schools company that school governing bodies could invest in – 75% of the shares are held by schools, the rest by the directors. They put together a business plan and the restaurant owner drew up menus with several mums who were keen on cooking. Then they hired a consultant who'd worked in school meals management to help prepare their tender to the LEA.

When they heard they'd won the contract in April 2006, it was all systems go: they needed to get the company up and running by September. They sold shares to the 21 schools and applied for a loan from the Local Investment Fund

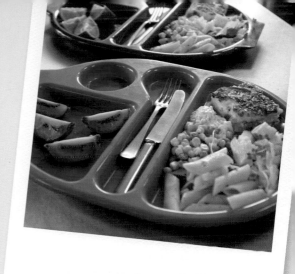

(www.lif.org.uk), which provides loans for social and community enterprises that wouldn't normally get traditional funding. They took on an Operations Manager, Julia Hallett, and re-employed all the existing catering staff at the schools. To help them get used to a whole new way of working, the local further education college's catering faculty got involved and came into school and held tailor-made workshops for staff,

WITHIN WEEKS HARRY WAS COMING IN FROM SCHOOL SAYING: 'WHY CAN'T WE HAVE FOOD LIKE THIS AT HOME?'

basing them on the new menus. Stephanie says it has transformed the staff's working life. 'Before they were undervalued – now they're skilled cooks. All have gone on to complete NVQ training.'

Whole School Meals aims to buy locally, so all the meat comes from Rook the butchers, an east Kent family firm (except chicken, which is from Norfolk). And about 70% of the fruit and veg delivered has been grown in Kent.

All the menus have been nutritionally analysed and there are regular get-togethers with the children and the cooks to discuss what goes down well and to ask for new ideas. On a typical week the children enjoy things like roast pork with apple sauce, leek and potato pie, macaroni cheese, spaghetti bolognese and vegetable biriani, followed by pineapple upside-down cake or apple pie and custard.

When Harry heard his mum was taking over the school kitchens, his first response was to roll his eyes and say, 'There's no way I'm going to have school dinners.' Within a few weeks he was coming in from school and saying, 'Why can't we have food like this at home?'

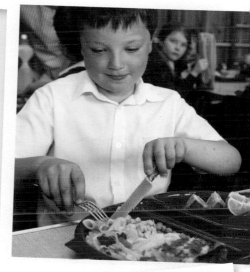

At the moment, Whole School Meals doesn't make a profit but the potential is there if they can boost the numbers of children having school dinners (currently around 30% of pupils do). A grant from the Lottery Wellbeing Fund will help – there are plans for after-school cookery clubs for children and parents, and food-theme days where chefs will come into school along with growers and producers.

To anyone contemplating setting up a similar company Stephanie says, 'Do it. It's a lot of work but it's worthwhile. What helped us was that we had a really clear vision from the outset. People could see what we were after.'

Visit www.wholeschoolmeals.co.uk for more information.

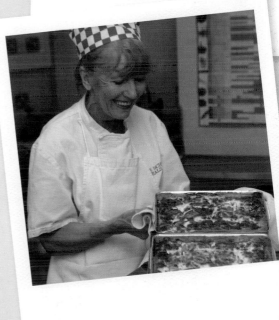

Spreading the word

Mick is a coach for the local football team that his son plays for. He soon realised that he had an influence not just on his son but on the other players too and wondered how he could use that to get the healthy-weight message across as well as coaching the game.

The 5 Simple Rules fit very well with a sports regime. Mick found that he could share the rules with his team quite easily, pointing out how football practice helped them towards the hour a day activity that makes up Rule 4. As an agent for change he also spread the word to the players' parents and to other coaches he met up with at matches.

More reasons to change

In 2003, a survey found that one third of 12-year-olds and half of 15-year-olds had had some kind of dental decay, which is linked to high sugar levels in food, especially in fizzy drinks and sweets eaten between meals. In 2000, research showed that half of adolescent girls weren't getting enough iron from their food and one fifth weren't getting enough calcium.

Activity in schools

What can you do if you feel your school isn't doing enough to help your child be active? The head teacher is probably making sure the school curriculum meets the minimum requirements for PE lessons but that won't be enough to fulfil a healthy-weight home goal of an hour's activity a day. This is where you can step in. Head teachers have a vast number of concerns to juggle and an agent for change can take some of the pressure off.

An ideal first step is to join the Parent, Teacher and Friends Association (PTFA) and get to know what the school's priorities are. Find out what grants are available in your area for after-school sports and coaching. Most sports clubs are run by volunteers and you don't have to be sporty yourself to set up a club. If you organise the basics then you can get in a professional coach to do the sporty bit.

In the wider world

Everyone has a part to play in tackling the rise in obesity, and the government is encouraging all sectors of society to get together – schools, doctors' surgeries, town planners, advertising and media, food and leisure industries – to help change the way we live. It's never been easier to get involved in all sorts of different ways.

For example, the National Institute for Health and Clinical Excellence (NICE) now has guidelines to help town planners and local transport authorities make the environment work for our health and against obesity.

How you can help run a sports club
→ Fundraising
→ Practical stuff like painting the club-house, clearing up the changing rooms after matches
→ Make or serve half-time refreshments
→ Ring round to see who is available for matches, who can drive the team to games
→ Do the accounts
→ Apply for grants

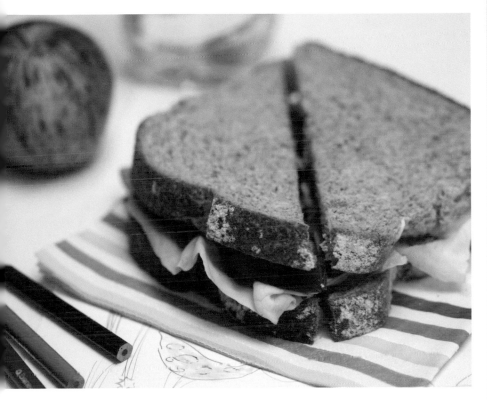

Getting to and from school

Carla wanted to build more activity into her children's lives and the ideal way would be for them to cycle to school. But both she and her husband were worried about one particular road where cars regularly broke the speed limit.

As an agent for change the first thing Carla did was to ask other parents whether they shared her concerns and whether they'd be prepared to lend a hand campaigning. Then she approached the school to see if they had a travel plan in place. The head teacher was keen to develop a plan and asked Carla if she could set things in motion. This was a big commitment with lots of elements. Her first job was to get the pupils involved, which she did by asking them to conduct a travel survey as part of their geography lesson. This gave her a clear picture of all the different ways children travelled to school. She also had to liaise with the school travel plan adviser at the local council. In the end Carla helped set up a 'cycle train' where groups of children cycle to and from school under adult supervision.

Websites Carla found useful were www.schooltravelplan.org and www.school-run.org

It has all sorts of commonsense suggestions to benefit everyone and these are things that we can get involved with at a local level, depending on what's happening where we live. NICE guidelines include closing off streets to cars to encourage people to walk, creating safe routes to school by using speed bumps to slow cars on school routes, improving footpaths, adding cycle lanes. These are all things that, as agents for change, we can campaign for. We can lobby for our public open spaces and parks to be well-maintained, well-lit, inviting places people that want to go to, and to ensure they are easily accessible on foot or by bike – or public transport.

New buildings such as hospitals, schools and shopping centres should be easily accessible by bike and on foot; they should have prominent well-lit staircases to tempt people to take the stairs, not the lift. School playgrounds need redesigning to encourage activity, with areas marked out for hopscotch or tag, for example, and new active climbing equipment. We can back up these ideas by adding our voices to the debate.

As an agent for change you can easily start the ball rolling by raising funds via the PTFA.

part 3
making it
work
for your family

different families have different needs

Creating a healthy-weight home is within every family's reach, but some of us will find it more of a challenge. Here we look at strategies to help different types of family meet their own specific goals.

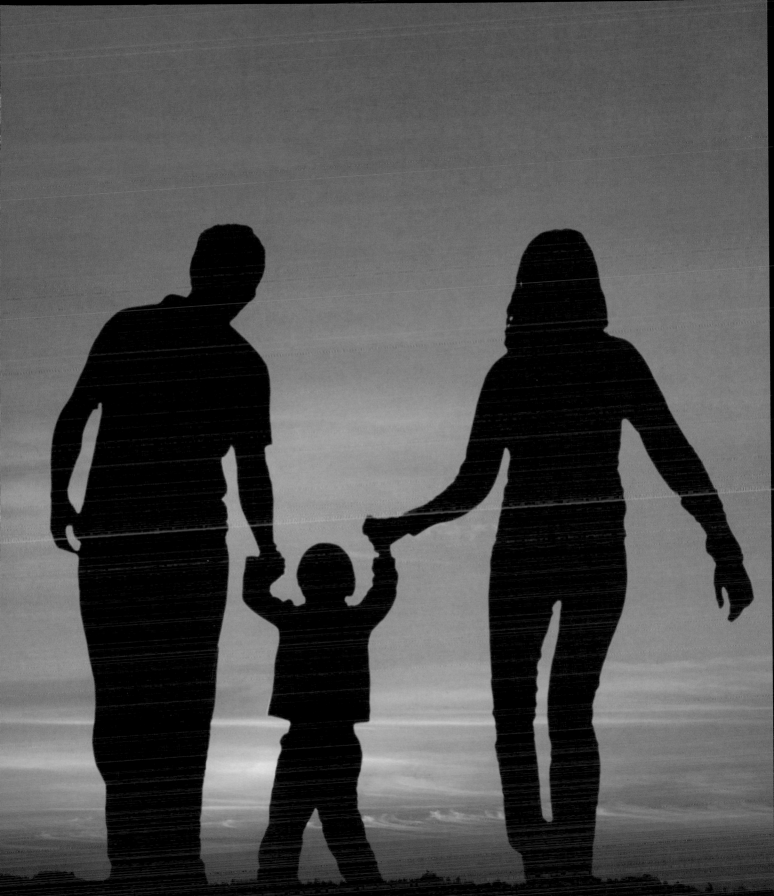

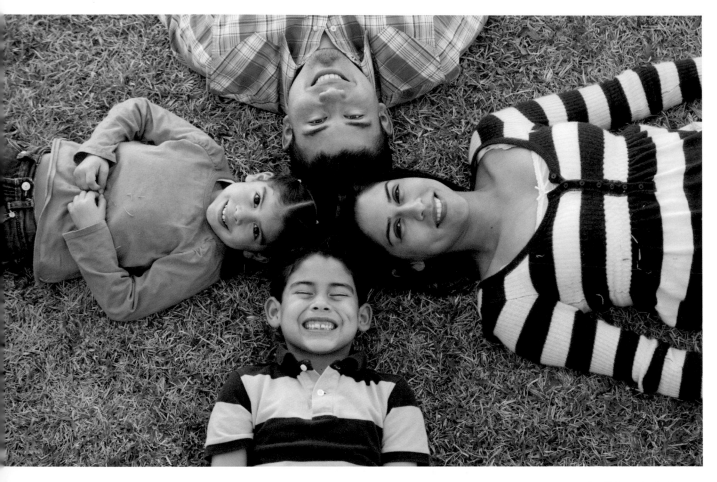

Different kinds of families

The term 'family' covers a range of situations: some families are split, with the children spending time in different households; others are a blend of two families coming together with complex combinations of step-siblings and new babies. Many families have a child with a physical or mental disability or with health problems. Regardless of how you define your family, you can still make your home a healthy-weight home. All you need are the 5 Simple Rules plus the agreement of all adults in the family to be positive role models, providers, enforcers, protectors and agents for change.

Children with disabilities

Experts stress that while a healthy (or healthier) body weight is a desirable goal for a child with special needs, it has to be seen as part of the broader picture and fit in with the child's other aims, which might include: encouraging activity; developing social skills; learning positive eating habits; and developing their potential.

Togetherness is vital

All children are affected by the contacts they have with other people, both in the home and outside it. Research shows that parents of a special-needs child can become upset if they think their child is being picked on or is not being respected by others. They can also feel isolated from other parents. The source of these feelings is obvious. For special-needs children to join in with everyday activities means meticulous advance planning on the part of their parents – something which others all too readily see as a hassle. It gets worse as the child gets older, when their peers often leave them out of their plans because it all gets too complicated for them to be included. Parents need to understand what is happening and give extra support, empathy and encouragement.

Research has shown that one way to boost the confidence of a special-needs child is to make sure the whole family sits down together for regular meals: it increases feelings of togetherness and helps the child feel less isolated – and reduces parents' stress levels.

Other ways of boosting family togetherness include making sure that both parents are involved in any therapy the child is having, which has also been shown to improve a child's progress. Parents of special-needs children also say that despite the increase in stress in their daily lives from coping with their child, one of the advantages it has is bringing the family closer together. Another is that the whole experience makes them far more thoughtful and sensitive to the needs of others, which in turn makes them especially effective agents for change.

Brothers and sisters of a special-needs child can also develop higher self-esteem, respect for other peoples' feelings and generally have a good attitude to life.

Unconventional families

Divorce is the biggest reason for the change in family structure. According to the Office for National Statistics, in 2005 more than 136,000 children under 16 were affected by their parents' divorcing.

Splitting up the household can have a noticeable effect on a child's routine, especially when it comes to eating and being active. In a single-parent family money is often tight, which affects the parent's ability to be a provider – of food and activity.

Parents often ask

Is there anything I can do to reduce my special-needs child's feelings of isolation?
The best way is to plan activities and then invite other children to join in, rather than sitting back and waiting for your child to be invited out. By doing this, you take responsibility for planning for special needs and remove the barrier that may have been making others reluctant to invite your child to parties and days out.

My working life just doesn't allow me to eat dinner every night with the children. Does that make me a bad parent?

Not at all. Family meals do not have to be dinner and they don't have to happen every day of the week. Even having breakfast together on Saturday morning or dinner on Sunday nights can make a difference.

On the positive side, however, establishing a new household can be the opportunity for a fresh start – and an ideal time to adopt the 5 Simple Rules. It's a chance to set new meal times, try new foods; it's an opportunity to limit screen time and introduce new activities. Moving to a new area means doing the grocery shopping at new shops and markets; there will be parks to explore, restaurants to try out and leisure centres offering different activities. Parents can introduce new rules and become better food and activity role models.

Whether it's the result of divorce or the death of a parent or for another reason, moving to

MAKING AS MUCH TIME AS POSSIBLE TO CREATE A HEALTHY-WEIGHT HOME CAN HELP IMPROVE A CHILD'S HEALTH

a new home has an impact on a child's psychological well-being. Separation from one parent can reduce the amount of time spent with that parent's extended family, for example. If that contact was positive and supportive, the child may feel abandoned. They may not talk about the stress of switching from a two-parent family to a one-parent family; instead they may

bottle it up inside. At the same time the child may develop a negative attitude to food and activity. Changes in behaviour should ring alarm bells – children with these symptoms are at greater risk of low self-esteem and of developing eating disorders. It's a good idea to get guidance and advice from an expert at this point. Chapter 13 has useful information on finding help.

Single parents

It can be tougher for single parents to create a healthy-weight home. For a start there's often less money coming in and they often have less time to focus on the 5 Simple Rules, such as cooking wholesome nutritious meals or finding time to be active during the day. Regardless of these obstacles, making as much time as possible to create a healthy-weight home is worth it and can help improve a child's health.

Togetherness makes a big difference. A survey of mothers and children aged 10-14 showed that family togetherness was the best predictor of healthy family habits. Other factors included family pride, confidence, self-control and a good support network in place.

Once again the simple fact of sitting down together to eat as a family promotes togetherness. Research has shown that families

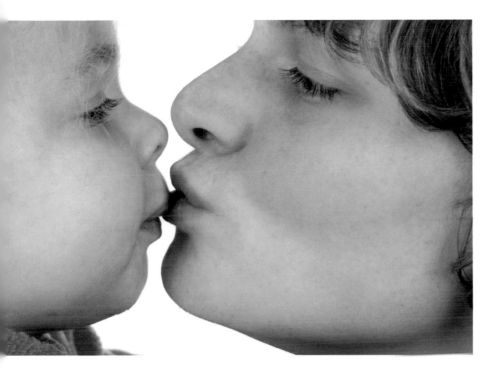

Parents often ask

Which is better, getting the children to follow a rule that my husband refuses to agree to, or not having the rule at all?

There are thousands of food and activity behaviours that you can change to create your healthy-weight home, so you can pick and choose which ones suit you and your family – it doesn't have to be all or nothing. Choosing those changes that your husband is willing to make and being consistent in following them is generally the best strategy.

who eat together improve their chances of good health. Meal times are the best time to be a food role model. Eating together can enhance the health and well-being of adolescents in the family. In one study, teenagers who frequently ate dinner with the family were less likely to smoke cigarettes or marijuana or to drink alcohol. They were also less likely to have low marks at school or to show signs of depression. Children who eat dinner with the family are also more likely to eat breakfast.

Getting everyone on board

In an ideal world every member of the family would be committed to creating a healthy-weight home

but, in practice, it's not unusual for one or more adults in the household to be unsupportive. In some cases they may feel that it's not important   for themselves or for their children. Or they may lack confidence in their ability to succeed; or they may just be unwilling to try. Whatever the reason, you'll have to work harder to find a way round the situation.

Differences of opinion between parents need to be avoided at all costs for the health and well-being of your children. Research shows that children with parents who argue a lot are more likely to have trouble with their own relationships with their parents. Conflict between parents can add to a child's feelings

Parents often ask

Sue and Andy liked to flop in front of the tv when they got home after work while five-year-old Emily preferred to play outside. But because she wanted to spend time with her parents she started coming in to sit with them and watch tv instead.

This is a classic example of how we parents influence our children – in this case in a negative way. Once Sue and Andy realised what was happening they knew they had to do something about it. They didn't need to go from one extreme to the other: they decided which tv programmes they couldn't bear to miss, then on the other days they played with Emily – nothing too strenuous, just the odd game of swingball or a gentle bike ride or even a bit of gardening. In wet weather they put on a favourite cd and danced instead. Being active for an hour a day isn't so daunting when you realise you don't have to join a club or go to a sports centre.

of insecurity and inability to cope. Children whose parents are getting divorced are at extra risk if their parents are at each other's throats all the time. High levels of family conflict create stress, which can be a trigger for a child to over-eat. Research suggests that a child whose parents argue constantly is likely to develop an eating disorder.

The art of compromising

When differences of opinion between parents are resolved in a positive way it can benefit the children: they develop confidence in their own emotions when they see grown ups listening to each other and working towards a common goal. When parents can't agree on the best way forward to creating a healthy-weight home, it's much better to compromise and stick with the changes that everyone is happy with rather than trying to go it alone or force someone to change.

In a split household, it goes without saying that the parent who spends most time looking after the children will have the greatest influence on changing family structure to create a healthy-weight home. Parenting style also makes a difference. An authoritarian or overly strict parent risks alienating the children from the whole idea of a healthy-weight home and they

may react by rebelling against the 5 Simple Rules. An overly permissive or hands-off parent is unlikely to encourage children to change their ways. The ideal parent is authoritative without being authoritarian: they're in charge and in control but don't throw their weight around.

Look after yourself

Our own health and well-being affects our children: if you're happy, your children will be too. And if they're happy, they'll adapt readily to changes in lifestyle. Now is the time to seek help if you're suffering from depression or feeling withdrawn – common reactions to divorce, separation or the death of a partner or close family member. If you don't deal with problems effectively you'll have a knock-on effect on your children. Girls are particularly at risk of developing weight issues when their mothers are depressed.

One of the best ways for parents to stay healthy is to follow the 5 Simple Rules, whether the children are around or not. If you need to lose weight, join a structured weight-loss programme such as Weight Watchers. Research shows that adults who've lost weight on the programme have a higher quality of life and are full of vitality. What are you waiting for?

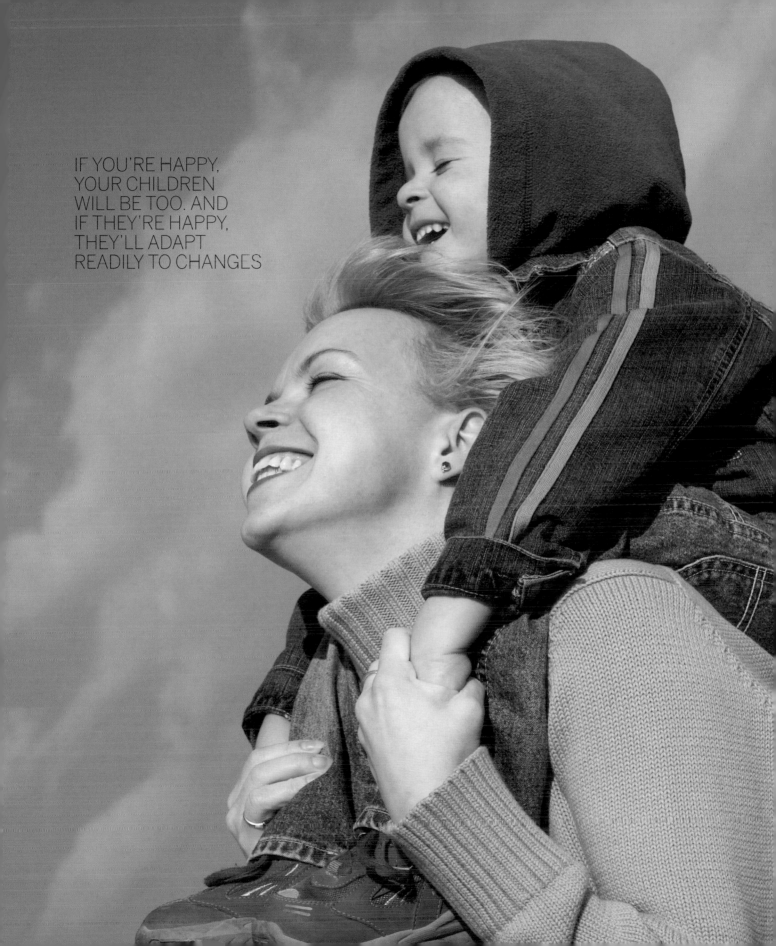

IF YOU'RE HAPPY,
YOUR CHILDREN
WILL BE TOO. AND
IF THEY'RE HAPPY,
THEY'LL ADAPT
READILY TO CHANGES

getting extra help

The 5 Simple Rules are the backbone of a healthy-weight home – but no one expects you to do it all alone. Even the government wants everyone to focus on a healthy lifestyle to reduce national obesity levels, so there's never been a better time to look for some extra help. Now is the time to get others involved: you'll find schools, doctors and other healthcare professionals ready and prepared to help. And don't forget the internet – it's a powerful research tool.

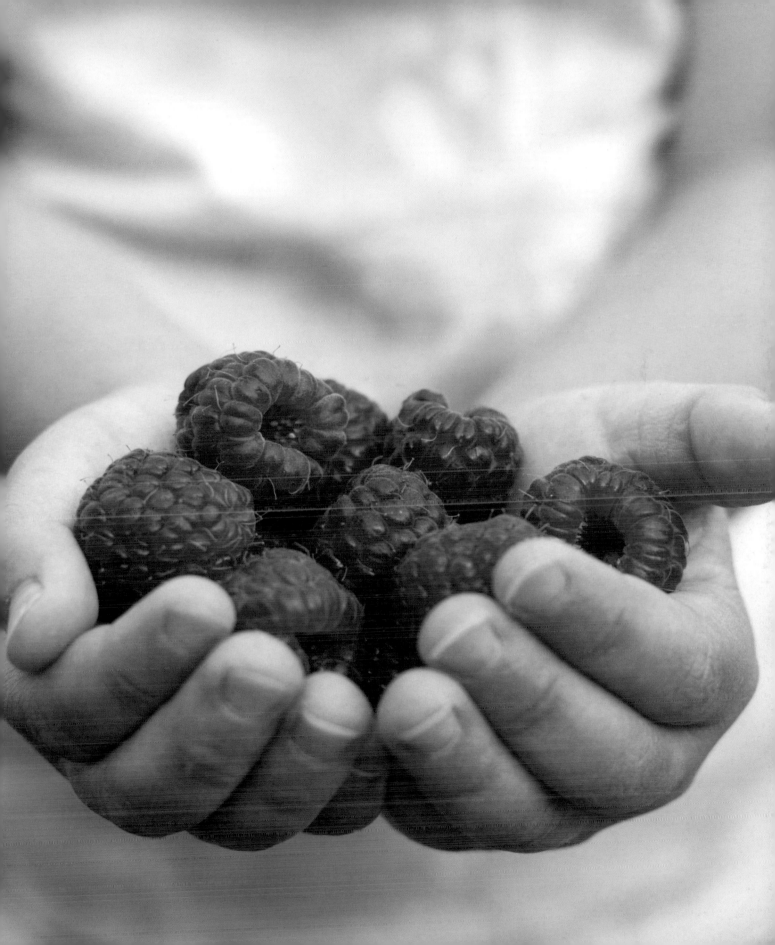

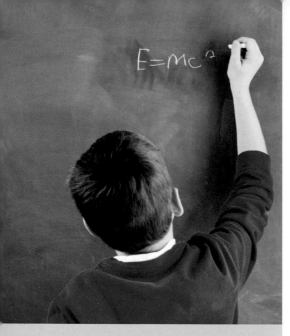

Schools and food

The parents section of the DirectGov website has clear information on school nutritional standards, as well as useful reminders on how to check whether your children qualify for free school meals. There's also up-to-date news on the latest food-related initiatives running in schools, such as the free fruit and veg schemes in primary schools. You can also use the site to find out who's in charge of school catering in your area. Visit www.direct.gov.uk/en/parents/ and click on 'Schools, learning and development'.

School support

Schools have never been in a better position to back up parents who are creating a healthy-weight home. With new standards aimed at improving school meals, free school fruit and veg for four- to six-year-olds, more PE on the curriculum and a big push to bring back cooking onto the timetable in secondary schools, you should find your local school very much in tune with everything you're trying to promote at home.

The National Child Measuring Programme is now well established in primary schools, meaning that your child's height and weight will be measured twice: when they first start primary school in reception class and before they leave in Year 6. Parents will be sent a letter detailing the results and asking them to enter them into an online BMI calculator to see for themselves whether their child is overweight. If you already know your child is overweight, there's no need to be nervous on their behalf about the process. Although it's carried out in school, it's done by trained professionals from your local Primary Care Trust and is done sensitively in a private room or screened-off area. Children will only be asked to take off their shoes and coat. And they will not be given the results to take home – or to compare in the playground.

If by any chance the school nurse or healthcare professional carrying out the measurements is worried about a child's weight, they will follow the local PCT's advice (which will vary from area to area) and take appropriate action.

Help from your GP

Primary Care Trusts – where your GP is based – have very different resources that vary across the country, so it's difficult to say what will be on offer. A city PCT may have a big budget and be able to afford its own dietician attached to the practice, whereas a small rural PCT wouldn't be able to justify the expense, for example. In most cases, the sort of help you can expect is regular monitoring of your child's weight by the practice nurse, or by the health visitor for very young children.

Your GP will also be able to refer you to a dietician to help you get started on looking at what your family is eating and how things can be improved. The dietician may work at your nearest hospital, but be prepared to go onto a waiting list before you get an appointment.

What's the difference between a dietician and a nutritionist?

A registered dietician will have trained to degree level, and will work mainly in hospitals and clinics, helping people to make informed decisions about food choices and lifestyle.

A nutritionist is a less precise term and not protected by law – so pretty much anyone can call themself a nutritionist and set up in business. Qualified nutritionists tend to work in a wider setting

A PSYCHOLOGIST CAN LOOK AT BEHAVIOURS THAT STOP A CHILD FROM ACHIEVING A HEALTHY WEIGHT

– not just in clinics and hospitals but in research and in the food industry or the media. They don't give individual advice unless they have a separate qualification in dietetics.

A child psychologist may be able to help

Your GP might decide that a psychologist would be able to help your overweight child. A child psychologist specialising in weight issues will be able to look at behaviours and feelings that may be stopping your child from achieving a healthy weight. Your GP may refer you to a psychologist attached to your local hospital or may refer you to your local Child and Adolescent Mental Health

Service. In some cases, your child's school may refer your child to a psychologist working within the local education authority. Again, it is likely that you will be put onto long waiting lists in both cases – up to six months is not uncommon and it can seem like a lifetime away. If you can't wait that long, there is another option: the British Psychological Society has a register of child psychologists working privately. To find one in your area, write or see the website:

The British Psychological Society
St Andrews House
48 Princess Road East
Leicester LE1 7DR
Tel: 0116 254 9568
www.bps.org.uk

Help with eating disorders

If you are worried that your child has developed an eating disorder, your first port of call should be your GP. If you need to find out more about the problem, have a look at the NHS website www.nhsdirect.nhs.uk/: you'll find useful links to self-help organisations and clinics that you can approach directly without a letter of referral from your GP. Click on the Health Encyclopaedia link and look up Eating Disorders in the A-Z index. Then click on Support Organisations on the right.

How to find your own dietician

If waiting lists are long and you can afford to pay to see a dietician privately, you can find a registered dietician working in your area by going online and visiting the British Dietetic Association's website at www.dietitiansunlimited.co.uk or you can write to:

Private Practice
The British Dietetic Association
5th Floor, Charles House
148/9 Great Charles Street
Queensway
Birmingham B3 3HT
Tel: 0121 200 8080

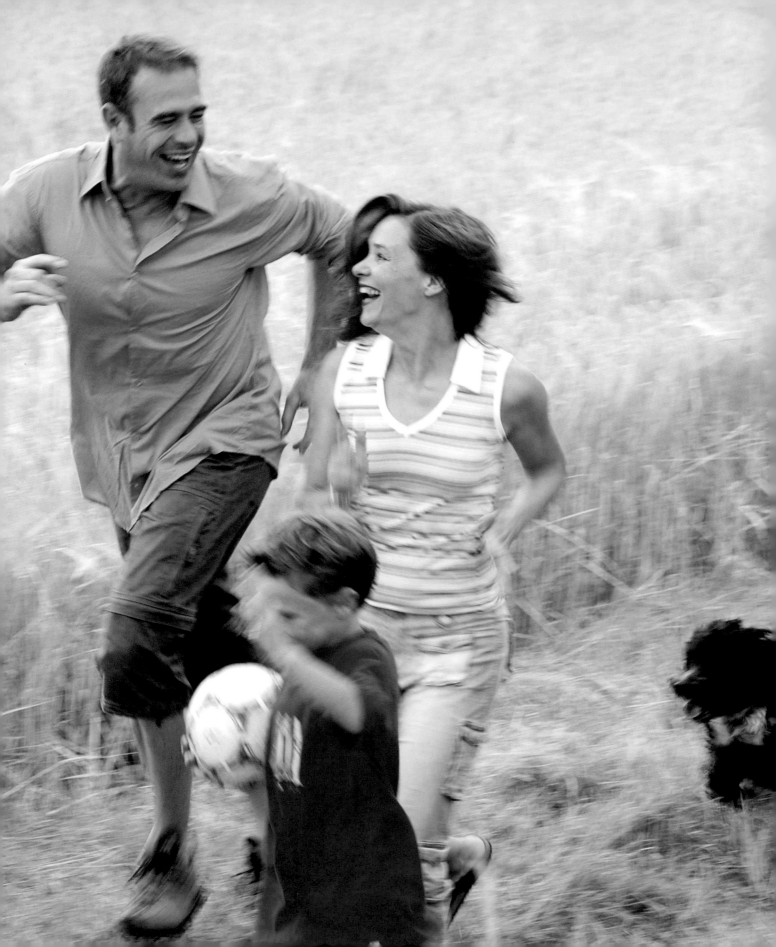

Help with getting fit

It often happens that a child is keen to get started on getting fitter but is put off by the thought of joining in with a group of peers – at least until they've made a bit of progress. This is when individual coaching with a fitness professional can help ease your child into an activity routine, giving them confidence and

INDIVIDUAL FITNESS COACHING CAN HELP IMPROVE YOUR CHILD'S CONFIDENCE AND ABILITY

helping them set realistic goals. This won't be a suitable option for younger children and you will have to confirm with any fitness professionals you contact which age groups they are qualified to work with.

Your local leisure centre or gym may have personal trainers you can book sessions with. Or you can search the National Register of Personal Trainers to find a qualified and insured trainer working in your area – see www.nrpt.co.uk or phone 0870 200 6010. Some trainers will come to your home to do a work out or you can arrange to meet them at the park or local pool. Or you may be lucky enough to find a trainer with their own private gym studio.

GET ONLINE!

→ **The Caroline Walker Trust** is a charity set up to improve health through good food. The trust regularly produces reports on nutritional guidelines for different groups of people, including children, people with learning disabilities and elderly people. The website has downloadable documents on topics such as 'Eating well for under 5s in childcare' and 'Eating well at school'. www.cwt.org.uk

→ **The School Food Trust** was established by the government's Department for Children, Schools and Families and the website is aimed at both schools and parents. It has lots of useful information on the nutrition-based food standards for schools plus ideas for healthy mid-morning snacks, a parents' forum and a case studies section where you can post your own school's experience of getting to grips with the new nutrition-based food standards and turning them into workable menus that pupils enjoy. Plus all the latest news, such as the debate on serving tea and coffee in secondary schools. www.schoolfoodtrust.org.uk

→ **The Food Standards Agency** website is brilliant for parents. It's clearly set out, easy to use and offers so much – from menu ideas for toddlers to Q&A sessions for teenagers. There's a whole section on food labelling – including traffic light labelling and definitions of all those baffling terms like 'best before' and 'use by'. It even has great ideas for packed lunches (useful if you've got stuck in a rut with ham sandwiches and an apple). The section on obesity has a handy BMI calculator. www.eatwell.gov.uk

part4
food
for all the family

healthy eating is fun

Wholesome foods are high in important nutrients like vitamins and minerals. They also tend to be lower in calories than less nutritious foods. For these reasons they should be the foundation of a healthy-weight home. But they're not just worthy, they're delicious too – as you'll see from the recipes in this chapter.

Wholesome foods supply children with the nutrients they need to grow, develop and stay healthy. Foods that are high in nutrients and lower in calories also help adults to meet their nutrition needs for health and well being without taking in too many calories.

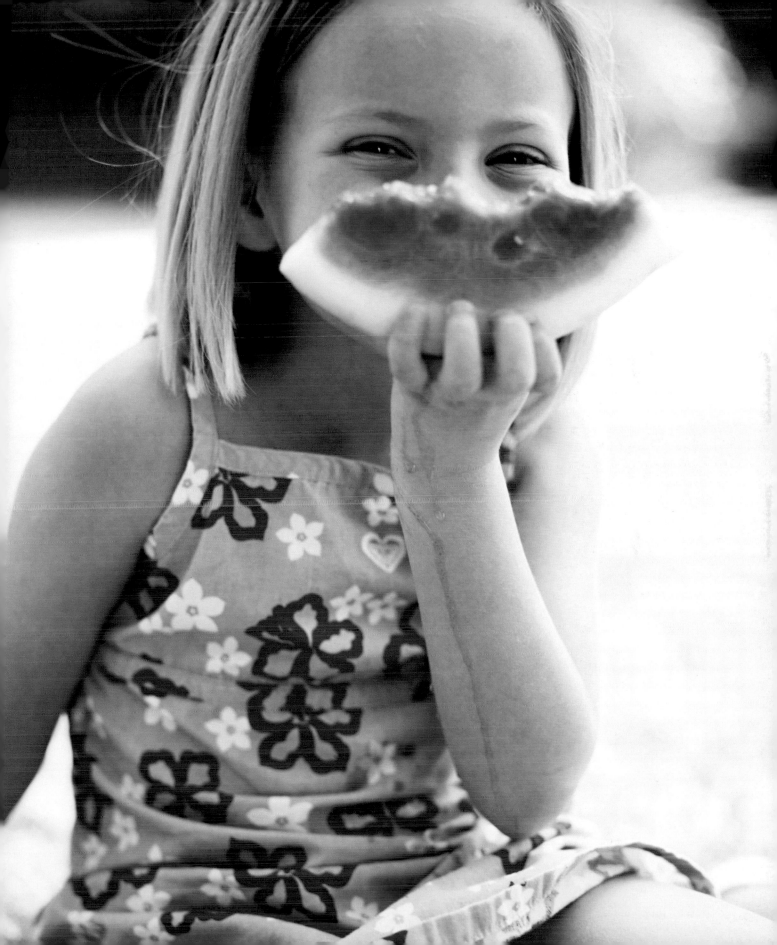

the wholesome

What are wholesome foods?

Wholegrains like wholemeal bread, wholewheat pasta, brown rice and high fibre cereals provide B vitamins, phytochemicals (beneficial plant compounds) – and fibre, which boosts feelings of fullness and helps the bowel function normally.

Fruit and vegetables provide a combination of vitamins and phytochemicals that no other type of food can match. They're filling because of their fibre and water content even though most don't have a lot of calories.

Proteins such as lean cuts of beef, lamb, pork and veal, along with skinless poultry, fish, eggs and meatless proteins – pulses, soy products and nuts – are necessary for general health and also make meals more satisfying. Many proteins are important sources of key vitamins and minerals.

Water, calorie-free drinks, low fat and fat-free milk are healthy choices and good alternatives to soft drinks and juices. Milk has the calcium and vitamin D that children's bones use to grow. Water and calorie-free drinks quench thirst without adding extra calories.

Healthy oils such as sunflower and olive oil, in small amounts, supply vitamin E.

Meat

Choose lean meat; trim any fat and throw away any fat that results from cooking.

Bacon, lean back
Beef
Gammon
Ham
Lamb
Mince – of any meat with 7% fat or less
Offal
Pork
Rabbit
Venison

NOT INCLUDED: Sausages, frankfurters, streaky bacon, burgers, processed meat and fatty meats e.g. luncheon meat, salami, pepperoni, corned beef.

Poultry

Choose lean poultry, remove the skin and throw away any fat that results from cooking.

Chicken
Turkey – including minced turkey

NOT INCLUDED:

Breaded and battered poultry products.

Fish & Shellfish

Any plain fish either fresh or frozen.

Tinned fish should be in water, brine or tomato sauce, not in oil.

NOT INCLUDED: Breaded and battered fish.

Vegetarian foods

Quorn mince, chunks, deli rashers, plain fillets
Tofu

NOT INCLUDED: Quorn burgers and sausages and other vegetarian burgers and sausages.

Eggs

Eggs, any type

Dairy

Cottage cheese, any type
Fromage frais, low fat
Low fat soft cheese
Quark

Soya milk
Yogurt, low fat or very low fat – any flavour
Skimmed milk – for those over 5 years old Children up to the age of 2 years old should have whole milk. Children between the ages of 2-5 years old can have semi-skimmed milk – please refer to your health visitor for extra advice on this.

NOT INCLUDED: Processed cheese spreads, full-fat soft cheeses and hard cheeses.

Fruit

Any fruit either fresh or frozen with no added sugar. Tinned fruit must be in water or juice and not syrup.

NOT INCLUDED: Fruit juices and dried fruit.

Vegetables

Any vegetables either fresh or frozen
Tinned vegetables must be in brine and

foods list

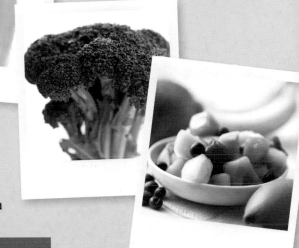

have no added sugar.
NOT INCLUDED: Frozen or tinned vegetables in sauces or with added flavourings.

Soups
Dried
Homemade with any Wholesome Food List ingredients
Restaurant made
Tinned
NOT INCLUDED: Creamy soups

Beans and pulses
Aduki
Baked (in tomato sauce)
Black eyed
Broad
Butter
Cannellini
Chick peas
Flageolet
Haricot
Kidney
Lentils, red, green or brown
Mixed pulses
Mung
Pinto
Soya
Yellow split peas

Bread
Wholegrain bread and rolls – any type
Reduced-calorie bread and rolls – any type

Breakfast cereals
Cereals must be eaten with skimmed milk (or milk appropriate for the age group) – not as dried cereal.
All-Bran
Bran Flakes
Corn Flakes
Porridge
Puffed Wheat
Rice Krispies
Shredded Wheat
Shreddies
Special K
Weetabix

Grains
Buckwheat
Bulgar wheat
Couscous
Crispbread, wholewheat
Millet
Noodles
Pearl barley
Polenta
Popcorn (air popped, fat free)
Quinoa

Rice – brown or wild
Rice noodles
Semolina
Wholewheat pasta

Drinks
Coffee
Diet drinks – any under 1 calorie per 100 ml
Soda water
Tea
Water or mineral water
NOT INCLUDED: Fruit juices and alcoholic drinks.

Oils
Olive
Rapeseed
Safflower
Sunflower
All above in small amounts e.g. 1-2 tsps.
Low fat cooking spray
NOT INCLUDED: Margarine, butter and other spreads.

Condiments, sauces and dressings
Apple sauce (unsweetened)
Artificial sweetener
Baking powder
Beef extract
Bicarbonate of soda

Capers
Cream of tartar
Curry powder
Fat- or oil-free dressings
Gelatine
Gravy granules
Herbs – fresh or dried
Lemon juice
Marmite
Mint sauce
Mustard
Passata
Pepper
Salsa
Soy sauce
Spices – fresh or dried
Stock cubes – any type
Sugar-free jelly
Tabasco pepper sauce
Teriyaki sauce
Thai fish sauce
Tomato purée
Vanilla essence
Vinegar
Wasabi paste
Worcestershire sauce
Yeast extract

great breakfasts

Research shows that children who eat breakfast are less likely to be overweight than children who don't. So make sure they start the day right with these easy recipes that make a change from everyday cereal and toast.

BREAKFAST OMELETTE

Save on the washing up with this one-pan version of a cooked breakfast.

Takes 10 minutes ■ Serves 1

low fat cooking spray
80 g (3 oz) button mushrooms, quartered
5 cherry tomatoes, halved
2 medium eggs
freshly ground black pepper

1 Lightly coat a non stick frying pan with low fat cooking spray and cook the mushrooms for 2 minutes, stirring gently, then add the cherry tomatoes.
2 Beat the eggs with 1 tablespoon water and seasoning, then pour into the pan. Tip the pan from side to side to spread the egg around, then cook gently for 1½–2 minutes, or until set to your liking. Carefully fold over and serve on a warmed plate.

OVERNIGHT MUESLI

Oats make for a great breakfast as they provide slow-release energy throughout the morning.

Takes 5 minutes + overnight soaking ■ Serves 2

60 g (2 oz) porridge oats
1 apple, cored and grated coarsely
250 ml (9 fl oz) skimmed milk
to serve
2 heaped tablespoons 0% fat Greek yogurt
80 g (3 oz) fresh blueberries

1 Place the oats in a bowl or plastic container, stir in the apple and milk, cover and leave to soak and soften overnight in the fridge.
2 In the morning, top each bowlful with a heaped tablespoon of yogurt and the blueberries.

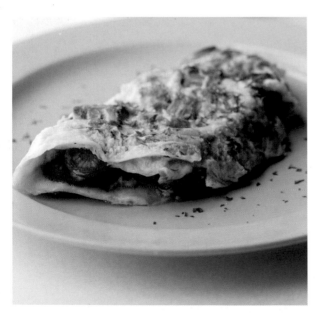

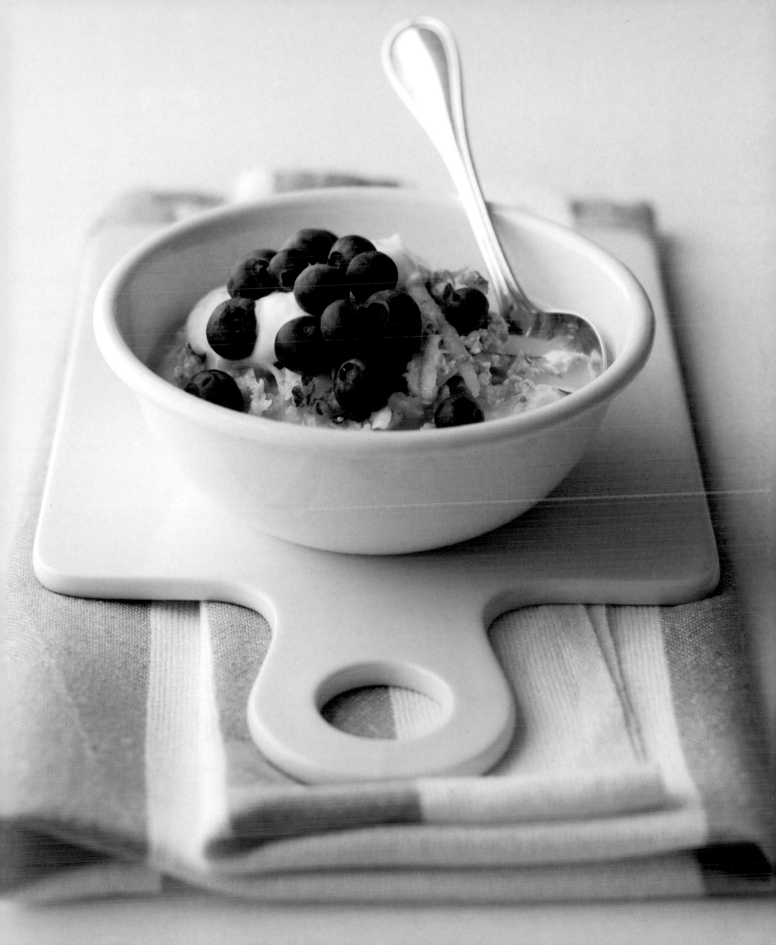

kids in the kitchen

The best way to get children to understand food is to get them involved in preparation. Here are some easy recipes they will have fun making.

TRIPLE DECKER LOLLY

Takes 10 minutes + 5½ hours freezing ■ Makes 6

150 g (5½ oz) fresh strawberries, hulled
2 x 100 g pots of low fat cherry layered fromage frais
1 x 120 g pot of low fat apricot yogurt
75 g (2¾ oz) fresh raspberries

1 Put the strawberries in a food processor or use a hand blender to whiz until puréed. Pass through a sieve to remove the pips. Set aside.
2 Mix together both pots of fromage frais and apricot yogurt. Set out 6 x 100 ml (3½ fl oz) lolly moulds and sticks. Put a spoonful of fromage frais mixture into the bottom of each lolly mould, then add a few raspberries, a lolly stick and freeze for 1 hour.
3 Remove from the freezer and pour over a little strawberry purée and freeze for a further 30 minutes. Repeat the layers again, using up the yogurt, raspberries and purée. Freeze for a final 4 hours or until frozen.

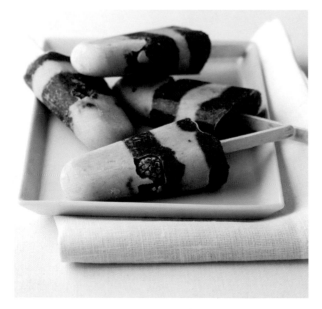

TEXMEX TORTILLA

Takes 20 minutes ■ Serves 2

low fat cooking spray
1 small onion, chopped roughly
1 red and 1 green pepper, chopped roughly
2 garlic cloves, crushed
pinch crushed dried chillies
½ teaspoon ground cumin
4 medium eggs
freshly ground black pepper
2 heaped tablespoons chopped fresh coriander

1 Lightly coat a non stick frying pan with low fat cooking spray. Fry the onion and peppers for 5 minutes until browned, then stir in the garlic, chilli flakes and cumin. Cover and cook for 2 minutes.
2 Preheat the grill.
3 Beat the eggs with seasoning and stir in the coriander. Pour over the vegetables and reduce the heat. Cook until the bottom of the tortilla is set.
4 Place the pan under the grill for 2 minutes to finish off the top, then serve, cut into wedges.

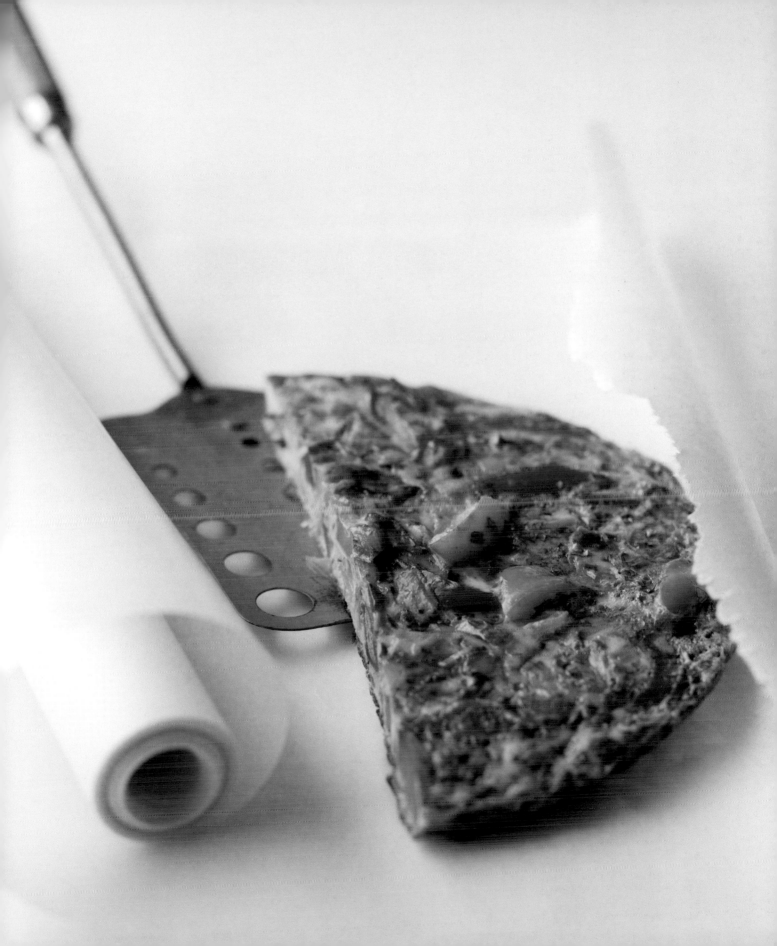

mid-week meals

It's not easy to be imaginative and health conscious every day of the week. When time is tight and your budget is stretched, you need evening meals that are quick and simple – and made from wholesome ingredients. A tall order? Not if you follow these recipes.

GRILLED SALMON WITH STIR FRY VEG

Takes 45 minutes ■ Serves 2

200 g (7 oz) brown rice
2.5 cm (1 inch) piece fresh root ginger, peeled and grated finely
1 garlic clove, crushed
4 tablespoons soy sauce
2 x 150 g (5½ oz) salmon fillets
low fat cooking spray
4 spring onions, sliced
200 g (7 oz) cabbage, shredded and washed
200 g (7 oz) cauliflower, cut into small florets
100 ml (3½ fl oz) vegetable stock

1 Cook the rice, following the packet instructions.
2 Meanwhile, in a small bowl, mix together the ginger, garlic and 2 tablespoons of the soy sauce. Place the salmon fillets on a plate and pour over the sauce. Place in the fridge.
3 Spray a large non stick frying pan or wok with low fat cooking spray and place on a high heat.
4 Toss all the vegetables together in the pan or wok, until browned on the edges, about 3–4 minutes. Add the stock, remaining soy sauce and stir fry for a few more minutes. Keep warm while you cook the salmon.
5 Remove the salmon from the fridge and place on a grill pan. Scrape any remaining ginger, garlic and soy from the plate into the wok and stir into the vegetables. Cook the salmon under a medium grill for 3–4 minutes on each side, or until just cooked through.
6 Drain the cooked brown rice and serve it with the salmon on a bed of stir fry vegetables.
Variation If you like chillies, try adding a fresh chopped chilli to the stir fried vegetables.

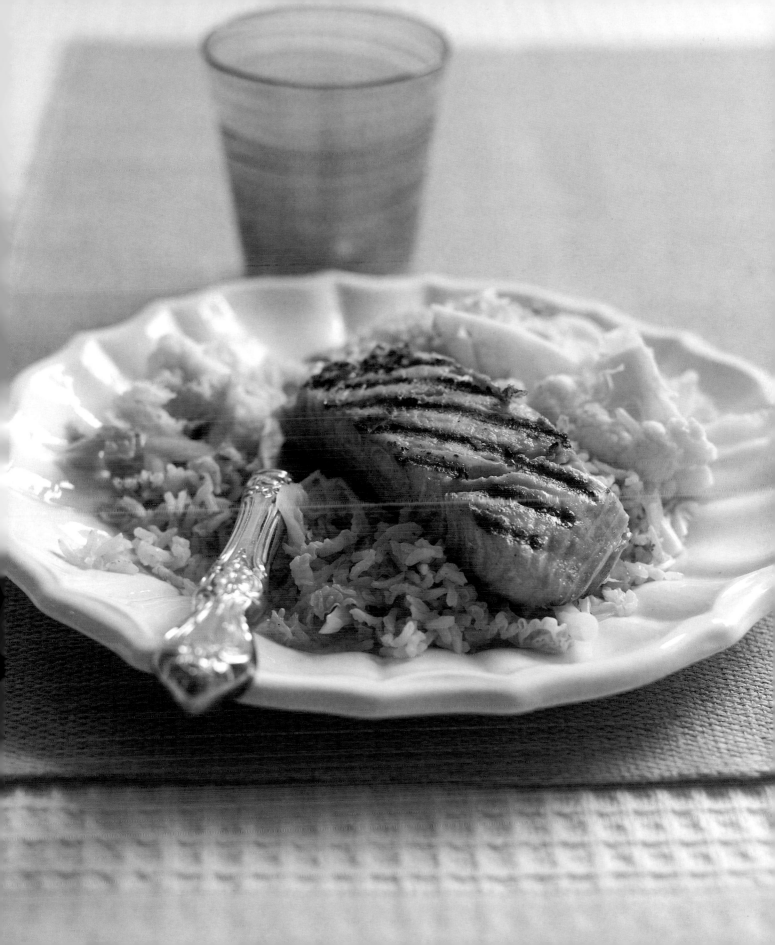

CHINESE CHICKEN

Takes 30 minutes ■ Serves 4

**4 x 150 g (5½ oz) skinless boneless chicken breasts, cut
    into small chunks**
1 garlic clove, crushed
2.5 cm (1 inch) piece of fresh ginger, peeled and grated
2 tablespoons soy sauce
juice of ½ a lemon
low fat cooking spray
1 green pepper, deseeded and sliced
1 carrot, peeled and sliced finely
½ red chilli, deseeded and sliced finely
1 onion sliced
100 ml (3½ fl oz) white wine vinegar
2 tablespoons granulated artificial sweetener
100 ml (3½ fl oz) passata
2 spring onions, sliced finely

1 Put the chicken chunks in a non metallic bowl and
mix with garlic, ginger, 1 tablespoon soy sauce and
lemon juice.

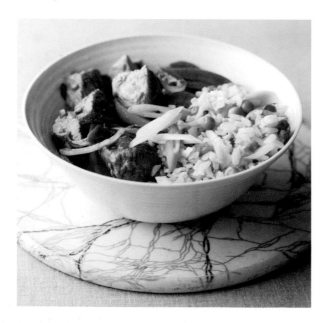

2 Heat a wok until hot. Spray with low fat cooking
spray and stir fry the chicken for 5 minutes until
starting to brown. Add the pepper, carrot, chilli and
onion and stir fry for a further 3 minutes.
3 Add the vinegar, sweetener, passata and remaining
soy sauce. Cook for 2 minutes until starting to thicken.
Sprinkle over the spring onions.
Serving suggestion serve with egg fried brown rice.

COWBOY PIE

This hearty dish is a delicious vegetarian take on
Shepherd's pie.

Takes 45 minutes ■ Serves 4

1 onion, chopped
low fat cooking spray
200 ml (7 fl oz) vegetable stock
350 g pack Quorn mince
420 g can low fat, low salt baked beans
230 g can chopped tomatoes
freshly ground black pepper
**750 g (1 lb 10 oz) potatoes, peeled and cut into 5 mm
    (¼ inch) slices**

1 Preheat the oven to Gas Mark 7/220°C/fan oven
200°C. Cook the onion in low fat cooking spray for 5
minutes until softened.
2 Stir in the Quorn mince, beans, chopped tomatoes
and stock, season, and simmer for 5 minutes, then
pour into a baking dish.
3 Add the sliced potatoes to a large pan of boiling
water. Stir so that they don't stick together and cook
them gently for 4 minutes or until tender.
4 Drain carefully and arrange on top of the mince.
Lightly mist with low fat cooking spray and bake for 25
minutes until the topping is golden and crisp.

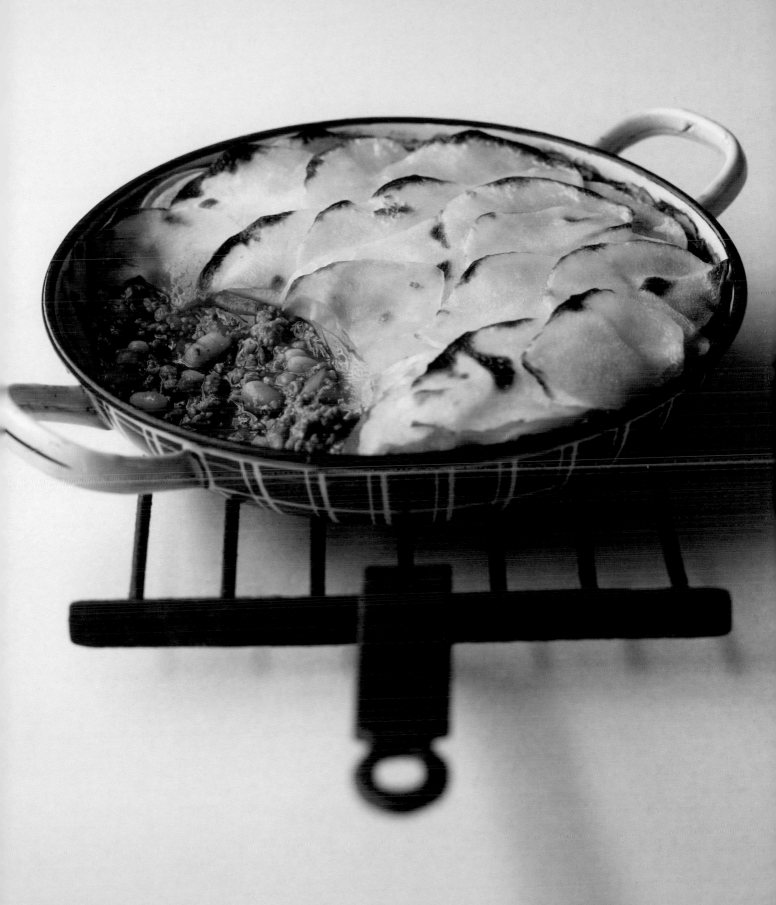

CHEAT'S SOUP

Takes 20 minutes ■ Serves 4

low fat cooking spray
1 onion, chopped finely
1 red pepper, deseeded and sliced
1 tablespoon mild or hot curry powder
1 x 700 g jar of passata with onion and garlic
50 g (1¾oz) fine green beans, trimmed and halved
300 ml (10 fl oz) hot beef stock
1 x 410 g can of chick peas, drained and rinsed
3 x 30 g (1¼ oz) slices of cooked lean roast beef, shredded
2 tablespoons chopped fresh coriander, plus extra to garnish

1 Heat a deep saucepan and spray with low fat cooking spray. Gently cook the onion and pepper for 5 minutes until softened. Add the curry powder, passata, green beans and beef stock and bring to the boil. Simmer for 5 minutes, stirring occasionally.

2 Add the beef to the soup, reserving a few shreddings for garnish. Add the chick peas. Cook for 1–2 minutes or until heated through. Check the seasoning; stir in the coriander.

3 Serve garnished with the reserved beef shreddings and the remaining coriander.

Vegetarian tip In step 2, replace the roast beef with 100 g (3½ oz) diced tofu. Spray a non stick frying pan with low fat cooking spray and fry the tofu until golden.

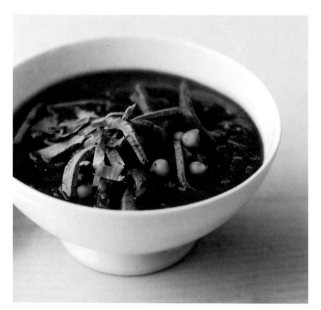

TURKEY WITH TOMATO AND CHICK PEA SAUCE

A delicious one-pot bake with turkey steaks cooked on top of an olive and garlic tomato sauce.

Takes 10 minutes to prepare, 25 minutes to cook ■ Serves 4

1 x 400 g can chopped tomatoes
1 x 410 g can chick peas, drained
30 g (1¼ oz) black olives in brine, drained and chopped
2 garlic cloves, crushed
2 teaspoons dried mixed herbs
½ chicken stock cube, dissolved in 150 ml (5 fl oz) hot water
4 x 110 g (4 oz) turkey breast steaks

1 Preheat the oven to Gas Mark 5/190°C/fan oven 170°C.

2 Mix together the tomatoes, chick peas, olives, garlic, herbs and stock. Pour into a shallow ovenproof dish or roasting tin.

3 Place the turkey steaks on top and bake for 25 minutes until the steaks are beginning to brown, and then serve.

Serving suggestions Serve with four jacket potatoes and steamed broccoli.

Tip Try this recipe with 4 x 125 g (4½oz) skinless boneless chicken breasts instead.

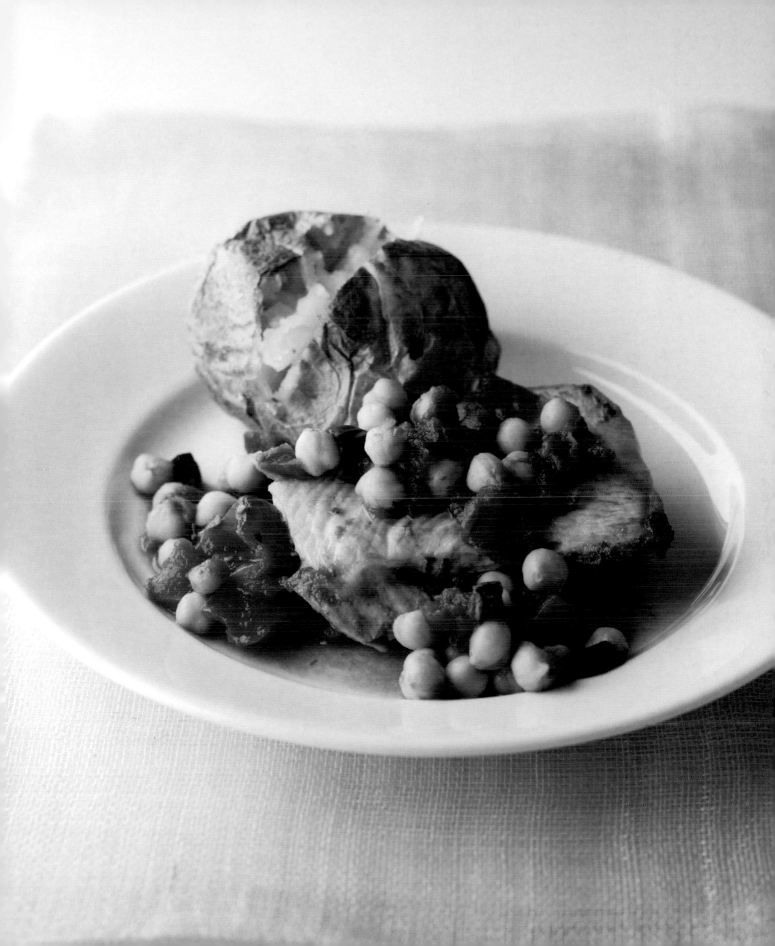

CHICKEN TIKKA LUNCHBOX

A satisfying portable lunch that makes a great change from everyday sandwiches.

Takes 15 minutes, plus 30 minutes marinating ■ Serves 1

for the chicken tikka
3 tablespoons low fat plain yogurt
1 teaspoon medium curry powder
1 teaspoon tomato purée
1 x 100 g (3½ oz) skinless chicken breast
for the salad
40 g (1½ oz) brown basmati rice
1 teaspoon chopped fresh mint or pinch dried mint
5 cm (2 inches) piece cucumber, diced
½ yellow pepper, deseeded and diced
freshly ground black pepper

1 Mix together the yogurt, curry powder and tomato purée. Add the chicken breast, turn to coat and marinate for 30 minutes.
2 Meanwhile cook the basmati rice in boiling water for

10 minutes or until tender. Rinse in cold water; drain.
3 Cook the chicken under a preheated grill for 10–12 minutes or until cooked through, turning half way through the cooking time. Cool and slice.
4 Tip the rice into a bowl with the mint, cucumber and yellow pepper and mix together.
5 Season to taste, then transfer to a lunchbox and top with chicken. Store in the fridge until needed.

SPICY VEGGIE CHILLI

Takes 20 minutes to prepare, 20 minutes to cook ■ Serves 2

low fat cooking spray
1 onion, chopped
2 garlic cloves, chopped
1 red chilli, deseeded and diced
75 g (2¾ oz) mushrooms, sliced
75 g (2¾oz) Quorn mince
1 x 400 g can chopped tomatoes
200 ml (7 fl oz) vegetable stock
1 teaspoon yeast extract
1 x 410 g can kidney beans, drained
to serve
2 tablespoons 0% fat Greek yogurt
1 tablespoon freshly chopped parsley
1 teaspoon smoked paprika

1 Lightly coat a lidded non stick frying pan with low fat cooking spray. Heat until hot.
2 Add the onion. Cook for 5 minutes. Add the garlic, chilli and mushrooms. Stir fry for 2 minutes.
3 Add the Quorn, tomatoes, stock and yeast extract. Bring to the boil, cover and simmer for 15 minutes. Add kidney beans and cook for a further 5 minutes.
4 Serve with a tablespoon of yogurt and a sprinkle of parsley and paprika.

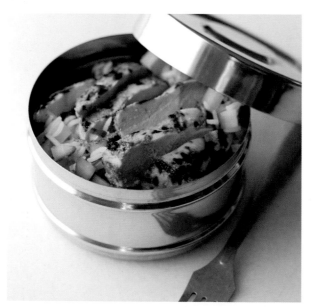

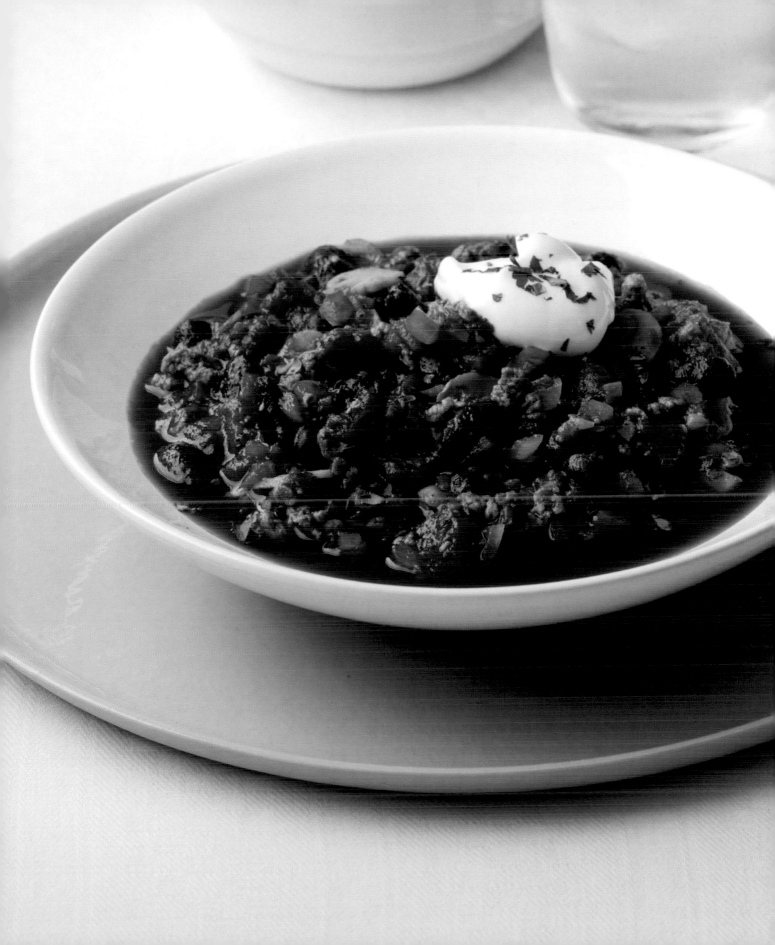

weekend family fare

When everyone is at home and relatives or friends are coming round, it's time to push the boat out a little. These delicious dishes look rich and sumptuous but are low on fat, sugar and salt. So get cooking and enjoy.

LAMB AND MINT BURGERS

Home-made burgers are not only delicious but, with lean meat, they are also low in fat.

Takes 30 minutes ■ Serves 4

for the burgers
low fat cooking spray
1 onion, diced finely
1 garlic clove, crushed
500 g (1 lb 2 oz) lean lamb mince
2 tablespoons freshly chopped fresh mint
freshly ground black pepper
for the mint relish
2 spring onions, sliced thinly
4 cm (1½ inch) piece cucumber, diced
2 tablespoons freshly chopped mint
1 apple, cored and diced
2 teaspoons lemon juice
to serve
a few tomato slices
a few Iceberg lettuce leaves

1 Lightly coat a frying pan with low fat cooking spray and heat until hot. Add the onion and garlic and cook gently for 7–10 minutes. Remove from the heat.
2 In a bowl, mix together the lamb, mint, cooked garlic and onion. Season. Form mixture into four burgers.
3 Spray the pan again with low fat cooking spray and heat until hot. Add the burgers and cook for 5–8 minutes on both sides until golden (or to your liking).
4 Meanwhile, to make the mint relish, combine all the ingredients in a bowl and set aside until required.
5 To serve, wrap the burgers in the Iceberg lettuce leaves, then top with a tomato slice and a spoonful of mint relish.
Tips Try these burgers with 500 g (1 lb 2 oz) minced pork, adding the zest of 1 orange to the meat instead of the mint. For the mint relish, try using the juice of a small orange instead of lemon juice.

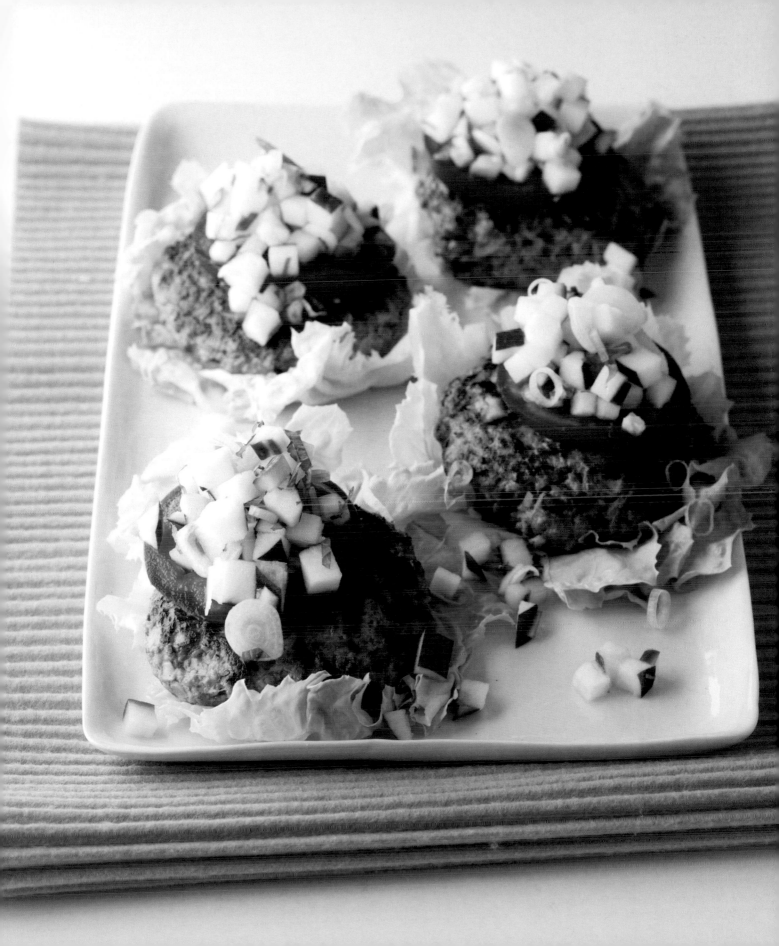

SWEET AND SOUR CHICKEN SKEWERS

These colourful skewers should prove a hit with friends and family of all ages.

Takes 25 minutes to prepare + marinating, 15 minutes to cook

■ Makes 12 skewers

1 x 432 g can pineapple rings in juice
2 teaspoons Chinese five spice powder
1 large garlic clove, crushed
2 tablespoons soy sauce
4 x 125 g (4½oz) skinless chicken breast fillets
2 red and 2 yellow peppers, deseeded and quartered

1 Drain the juice from the canned pineapple into a non metallic bowl or dish. Stir in the Chinese five spice powder, the garlic and soy sauce.
2 Cut each chicken breast into 12 chunky pieces and add to the marinade. Cover and marinate for at least 30 minutes.
3 Cut each pineapple ring into eight pieces, then chop each pepper quarter into six chunky pieces. Thread four pieces each of coloured pepper, chicken and pineapple on to each of 12 skewers.
4 Cook under a preheated grill for 15 minutes, turning once, until cooked and slightly caramelised.

ROASTED RAGOUT WITH BORLOTTI BEANS

This is a very easy, all-in-one pan recipe.

Takes 10 minutes to prepare, 55 minutes to cook

■ Serves 4

1 small courgette, trimmed and cut into chunks
1 yellow pepper, deseeded and sliced
1 red pepper, deseeded and sliced
2 red onions, cut into wedges
4 garlic cloves, unpeeled
1 rosemary sprig
low fat cooking spray
10 tomatoes on the vine
1 x 410 g can borlotti beans, drained
150 ml (5 fl oz) vegetable stock
freshly ground black pepper
a handful of basil leaves, to garnish

1 Preheat the oven to Gas Mark 6/200°C/fan oven 180°C.
2 Place the courgette, peppers, onions, garlic and rosemary in a large roasting tin. Spray with low fat cooking spray and cook in the oven for 30 minutes until beginning to char.
3 Add the tomatoes and cook for a further 15 minutes until they are soft.
4 Stir in the borlotti beans and stock, splitting some of the tomatoes so that they form a sauce. Cover with foil and cook for a further 10 minutes until hot.
5 Season and garnish with basil leaves before serving.

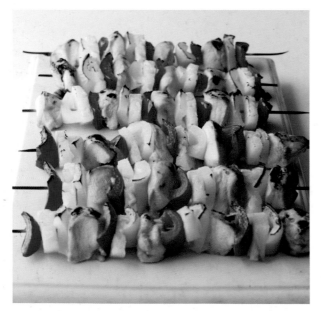

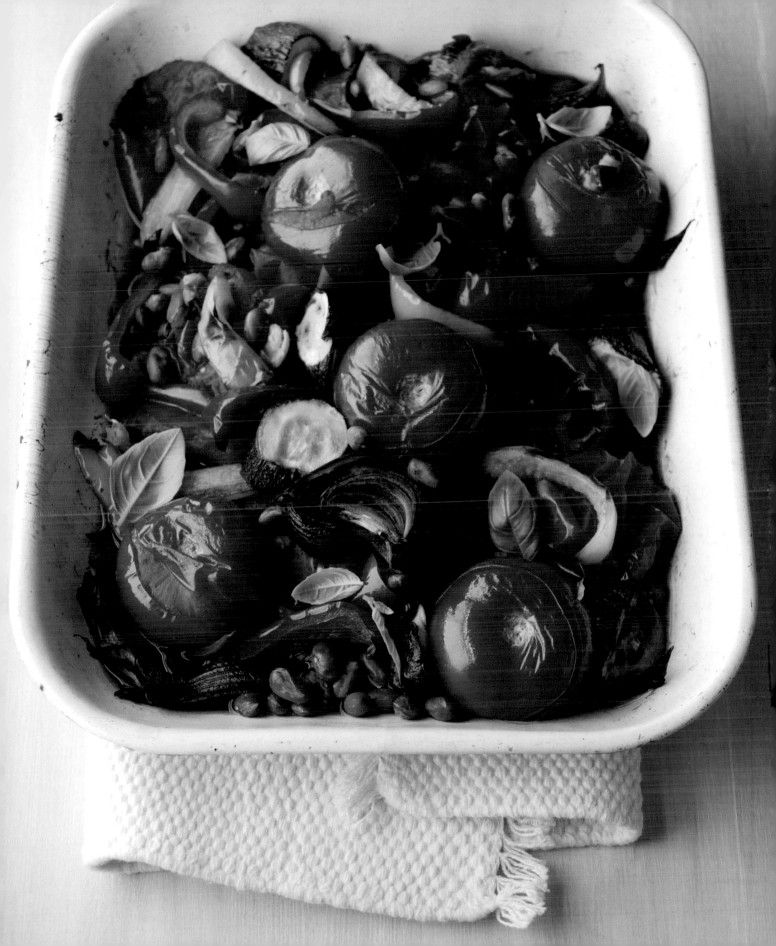

FRENCH ROAST CHICKEN WITH BOULANGÈRE POTATOES

The French roast their chickens breast-side down, which keeps the white meat deliciously moist and tender. The accompanying slow-cooked potato dish got its name because it used to be baked in the residual heat of the baker's oven, once all the daily bread was done.

Takes 15 minutes to prepare, 1 hour 15 minutes to cook
■ Serves 4

1.75 kg (4 lb) whole chicken
½ lemon
freshly ground black pepper
1 onion, thickly sliced
150 ml (5 fl oz) chicken stock
1 garlic clove, crushed
2 tablespoons freshly chopped tarragon
low fat cooking spray
for the boulangère potatoes
1 kg (2 lb 4 oz) potatoes, peeled and sliced thinly
1 onion, sliced thinly
300 ml (10 fl oz) skimmed milk
500 ml (18 fl oz) chicken stock
small bunch of watercress, to garnish (optional)

1 Preheat the oven to Gas Mark 5/190°C/fan oven 170°C.

2 Wipe the chicken inside and out with kitchen paper, tuck the lemon half inside and season with freshly ground black pepper. Place the sliced onion in a small roasting tin and sit the chicken on top, breast side down.

3 Roast for 45 minutes, then turn the chicken breast side up and cook for a further 20–30 minutes until the chicken is cooked. The juices should run clear when the thickest part of the leg is pierced.

4 As soon as the chicken is in the oven, layer the potato and onion slices in a baking dish, lightly greased with low fat cooking spray, seasoning as you go.

5 Pour the milk and chicken stock over the potatoes so that they are almost covered, then place a sheet of lightly greased foil on top.

6 Bake in the oven for 1–1½ hours, removing the foil for the last 10 minutes so that the potatoes can brown. The potatoes can be kept warm without spoiling if they are ready before the chicken.

7 When the chicken is ready, remove to a platter, cover with foil, and leave to rest for 10 minutes before carving. This will give a juicier, more moist chicken.

8 Place the roasting tin on the hob, using an oven glove to hold it, and add the stock, garlic and tarragon. Bring to a simmer, stirring to release the caramelised chicken juices from the tin, and bubble gently for 5 minutes.

8 Carve the chicken, removing the skin, and serve with the tarragon gravy and boulangère potatoes. Garnish with some sprigs of watercress if you wish.

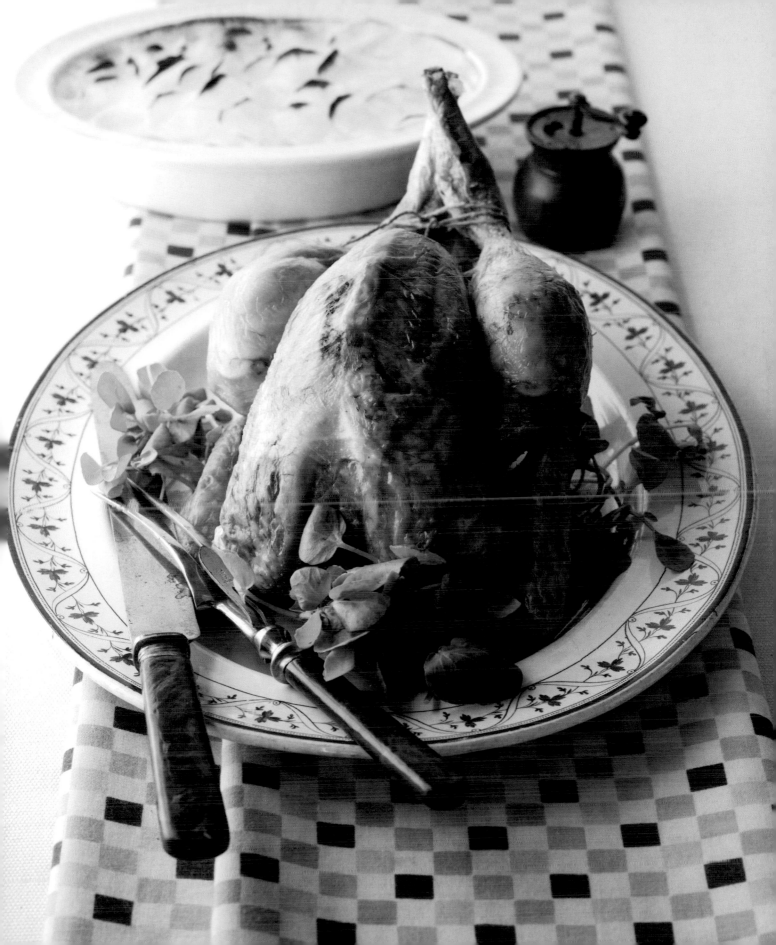

BLACKCURRANT MOUSSE

This recipe turns a sachet of sugar-free jelly into a stunning but simple dessert.

Takes 20 minutes to prepare + chilling ■ Serves 4

12 g sachet blackcurrant sugar-free jelly
juice ½ lemon
290 g can blackcurrants in juice
2 egg whites *
150 g (5½ oz) low fat plain yogurt

1 Sprinkle the sugar-free jelly crystals into 200 ml (7 fl oz) boiling water, stirring to dissolve.
2 Add the lemon juice and the juice from the can of blackcurrants. If necessary, add cold water to make the jelly up to 400 ml (14 fl oz). Pour into a large bowl and chill in the fridge for 30 minutes until the jelly is starting to thicken.
3 Whisk the egg whites to the soft peak stage. Stir the yogurt into the jelly, then fold in the egg whites.
4 Ladle into four ramekins; cover and chill for 3 hours or until set. To serve, spoon blackcurrants on top of each mousse.
***** If serving to toddlers then omit the egg whites - it still makes a delicious dessert.

MINT AND RASPBERRY JELLIES

These make a lovely, refreshing summer pudding and are particularly good for alfresco dining.

Takes 15 minutes + 1 hour chilling ■ Serves 4

10 mint leaves, torn
300 ml (10 fl oz) boiling water
1 sachet raspberry sugar-free jelly
125 g (4½ oz) raspberries, defrosted if frozen

1 Place the mint leaves in a jug and pour over the boiling water. Leave to infuse for 5 minutes.
2 Add the jelly to the jug and stir to dissolve. If it doesn't dissolve fully, microwave for a few seconds and stir again.
3 Reserve four raspberries and roughly crush the rest with a fork. Stir the crushed raspberries into the jelly and top up with cold water to make 600 ml (1 pint). Divide between four glasses. Cool and chill in the fridge for 1 hour until set.
4 Serve decorated with the reserved raspberries.
Tip Try this recipe using orange sugar-free jelly and fresh blueberries.

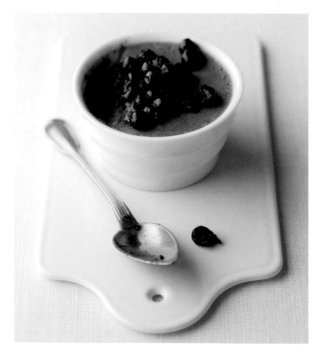

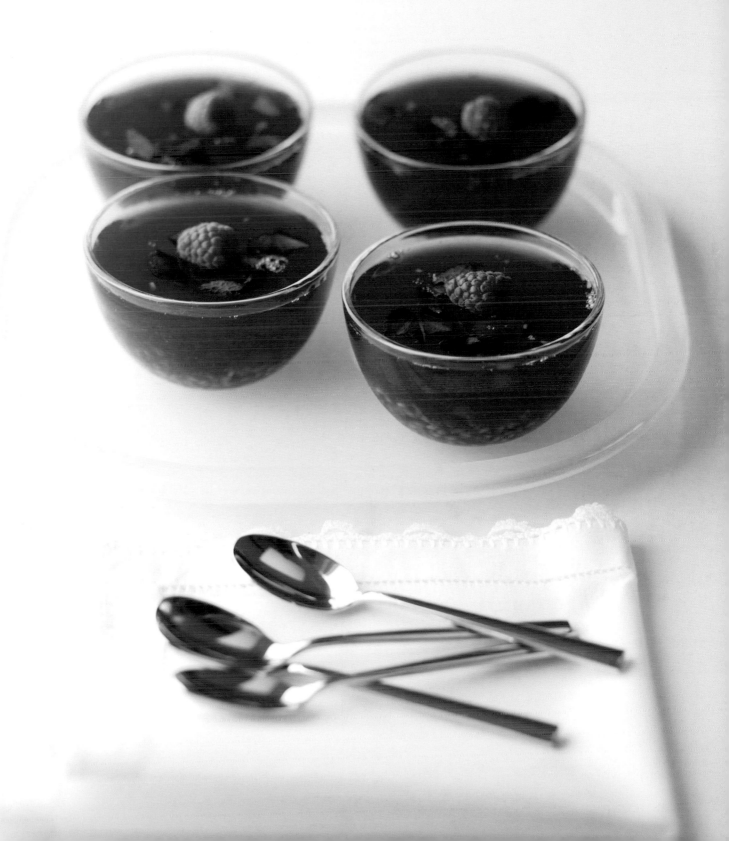

part 5
the family
action
plan

small steps to big changes

If you've read this book all the way through, then you've probably realised that to have healthy children you need to be a healthy parent. Being a good role model is hard work, but this book has many tools to help you succeed in your goal to have a healthy-weight home and healthy-weight children. In this chapter you will find charts and calendars that you can photocopy and get everyone involved in filling them in.

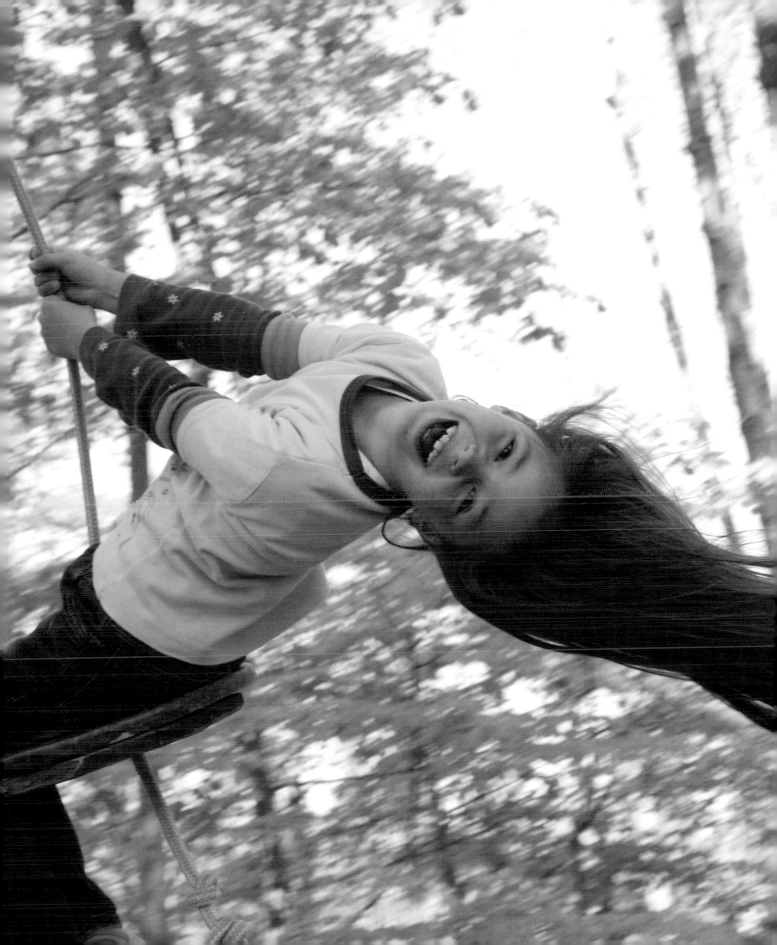

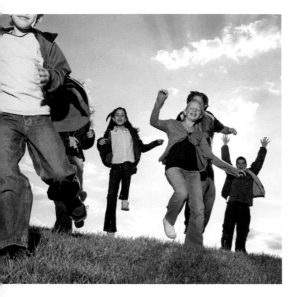

Setting goals, recording progress and offering rewards

Children love goals and incentives: if you put the relevant charts on the fridge door they will be able to see real progress each week. More activities and fewer screen hours combined with five-a-day fruit and vegetables and wholesome nutritious meals will all add up to real achievements. You can decide what the rewards are: gold stars, stickers or even a family treat to the cinema or a picnic – it's up to you.

Let's get physical

Get each member of the family to fill out a personal ACTIVITY LOG. For every day that they achieve 60 minutes of activity, give your children a sticker or a star – but don't deduct marks if they don't make it.

Strategies for success

➜ If it's at all practical, walk or cycle to school with your child once a week, instead of driving.

➜ Be an active adult. Take the stairs whenever possible. Walk the dog (if you have one), instead of just letting it out into the garden.

➜ Choose enjoyable activities: if you enjoy hiking, cycling and team sports, then your child will see that being active is fun.

➜ Get out and get active for at least half a day at the weekend.

➜ Encourage your children to play outside after school and before they start their homework.

➜ Make sure childcarers understand the importance of daily activity and the need to include it in your child's routine.

Screen time

Get every member of the family to fill out a SCREEN LOG. Each day that they spend less than two hours in front of a screen is an achievement. Give out stickers or stars that can build up into a reward.

Strategies for success

➜ Keep tvs, computers and video games (including handheld) out of the bedrooms.

➜ Monitor how long your child spends on non-homework screen time – chat rooms, online games and social networking sites – it all adds up.

➜ Get children to play for at least 30 minutes before homework – it'll give them a mental break and help meet daily activity requirements.

➜ Prepare meals as a family rather than leaving it all to one person while others are taking it easy sitting in front of the tv.

➜ Get everyone involved in other family activities, such as board games for indoors or garden games like quoits or swingball.

Family calendar

Fill in the FAMILY CALENDAR with activities that the whole family can do together – swimming, walking, biking, shopping. Write the number of minutes in the box and see if you can increase them each month. Keep all the charts on a noticeboard or on the fridge.

Strategies for success

➜ Keep a rucksack with Frisbee, bats, balls, skipping ropes, kite, etc, by the back door or in the car boot so you don't waste time searching for equipment before you go out.

➜ Keep up-to-date information leaflets on sports centres, leisure centres, swimming pools, etc, on a noticeboard or on the fridge.

➜ Have a family discussion so that everyone can make suggestions on activities you will all enjoy.

personal activity log

Stick a star ★ on each box for every 60 minutes of activity you achieve

my name ....

my goal is .... hours of weekly physical activity

	playtime with family or friends	movement in my daily routine	activity at school	structured physical activity	total
monday					
tuesday					
wednesday					
thursday					
friday					
saturday					
sunday					

screen log

my name ....

I estimate that I have _____ hours of weekly screen time

	television	computer	video games	total
monday				
tuesday				
wednesday				
thursday				
friday				
saturday				
sunday				

family calendar

family activities for the month of _____

fill in the date in each white box, and write in all your family activities and how long you spend doing them

monday	tuesday	wednesday	thursday	friday	saturday	sunday

part 6

references sources & index

references and sources

Chapter 1 What is a healthy-weight home?

Flodmark C-E, Lissau I, Moreno LA, Pietrobelli A, Widhalm K. New insights into the field of children and adolescents' obesity. *Int J Obes* 2004;28:1189-96.

Health Survey for England 2005.

Institute of Medicine of the National Academies. *Preventing Childhood Obesity: Health in the Balance.* Washington, D.C.: The National Academies Press, 2005.

Iwata F, Hara M, Okada T, Harada K, Li S. Body fat ratios in urban Chinese children. *Pediatr Int.* 2003;45:190-2.

Lissau I, Overpeck MD, Ruan WJ, Due P, Holstein BE, Hediger ML. Health Behaviour in School-Aged Children Obesity Working Group. Body mass index and overweight in adolescents in 13 European countries, Israel, and the United States. *Arch Pediatr Adolesc Med.* 2004;158:27-33.

Obesity – the new tobacco. Mintel 2006 p11.

Ogden CL, Flegal KM, Carroll MD, Johnson CL. Prevalence and trends in overweight among US children and adolescents, 1999–2000. *JAMA.* 2002;288:1728-32.

Prevalence of Overweight among Children and Adolescents: United States, 1999–2002. Centers for Disease Control and Prevention, National Center for Health Statistics. Accessed online May 4, 2005, at www.cdc. gov/nchs/products/pubs/pubd/hestats/ overwght99.htm.

Reducing and Preventing Obesity, everything must change. Royal College of Physicians 2004.

Survey on Childhood Obesity. Department of Health 2000.

Chapter 2 How to be an effective parent

Adams Larsen M, Tentis E. The art and science of disciplining children. *Pediatr Clin North Am.* 2003;50:817-40.

American Academy of Pediatrics. Family pediatrics: report of the Task Force on the Family. *Pediatrics.* 2003;1541-71. Accessed online April 30, 2005, at www.pediatrics. org/cgi/content/full/111/6/S1/1541.

American Heritage Dictionary of the English Language, Fourth Edition. New York: Houghton Mifflin Company, 2003.

Barlow J, Underdown A. Promoting the social and emotional health of children: where to now? *J R Soc Health.* 2005;125:64-70.

Barlow SE, Dietz W, Jr, Obesity evaluation and treatment: expert committee recommendations. *Pediatrics.* 1998;102:e29

Birch LL. Development of food acceptance patterns in the first years of life. *Proc Nutr Soc.* 1998;57:617-24.

Birch LL, Davison KK. Family environmental factors influencing the developing behavioral controls of food intake and childhood over-weight. *Ped Clin N Am.* 2001;48:893-907.

Cathey M, Gaylord N. Picky eating: a toddler's continuing approach to mealtime. *Pediatr Nurs.* 2004;30:101-7.

Fox KR. Childhood obesity and the role of physical activity. *J R Soc Health.* 2004;124:34-9.

Golan M, Weizman A. Familial approach to the treatment of childhood obesity: conceptual mode. *J Nutr Educ.* 2001;33:102-7.

Henze C, Plaza CI. Public health issue brief: physical education: year end report–2004. *Issue Brief Health Policy Track Serv.* 2004;1-16.

Hertzler AA. Children's food patterns—a review: II. Family and group behavior. *J Am Diet Assoc.* 1983;83:555-60.

Hertzler AA. Obesity—impact of the family. *J Am Diet Assoc.* 1981;79:525-30.

Hood VL, Kelly B, Martinez C, Shuman S, Secker-Walker R. A Native American community initiative to prevent diabetes. *Ethn Health.* 1997;2:277-85.

Kalb LM, Loeber R. Child disobedience and noncompliance: a review. *Pediatrics.* 2003;111:641-52.

Kolliker M. Ontogeny in the family. *Behav Genet.* 2005;35:7-18.

Licence K. Promoting and protecting the health of children and young people. *Child Care Health Dev.* 2004;30:623-35.

Longjohn MM. Chicago project uses ecological approach to obesity prevention. *Pediatr Ann.* 2004;33:55-7, 62-3.

McBean LD, Miller GD. Enhancing the nutrition of America's youth. *J Am Coll Nutr.*

1999;18:563–71.

McCaffree J. Childhood eating patterns: the roles parents play. J Am Diet Assoc. 2003;103:1587.

Moore H, Nelson P, Marshall J, Cooper M, Zambas H, Brewster K, Atkin K. Laying foundations for health: food provision for under 5s in day care. Appetite. 2005;44:207–13.

Moore LL, Lombardi DA, White MJ, Campbell JL, Oliveria SA, Ellison RC. Influence of parents' physical activity levels on activity levels of young children. J Pediatr. 1991;118:215–9.

Position of the American Dietetic Association: benchmarks for nutrition programs in child care settings. J Am Diet Assoc. 2005;105:979–86.

Weiss MR, Ebbeck V, Horn TS. Children's self-perceptions and sources of physical competence information: a cluster analysis. J Sport Exerc Psychol. 1997;19:52–70.

Chapter 3 The difference between adults and children

Chatterjee N, Blakely DE, Barton C. Perspectives on obesity and barriers to control from workers at a community center serving low-income Hispanic children and families. J Community Health Nurs. 2005;22:23–36.

Clarke WR, Lauer RM. Does childhood obesity track into adulthood? Crit Rev Food Sci Nutr. 1993;33:423–30.

Epstein LH. Family-based behavioural intervention for obese children. Int J Obes Relat Metab Disord. 1996;20:S14–21.

Institute of Medicine of the National Academies. Preventing Childhood Obesity: Health in the Balance. Washington, DC: The National Academies Press, 2005.

McLean N, Griffin S, Toney K, Hardeman W. Family involvement in weight control, weight maintenance and weight-loss interventions: a systematic review of randomised trials. Int J Obes Relat Metab Disord. 2003;27:987–1005.

Saxena R, Borzekowski DL, Rickert VI. Physical activity levels among urban adolescent females. J Pediatr Adolesc Gynecol. 2002;15:279–84

Wrotniak BH, Epstein LH, Paluch RA, Roemmich JN. Parent weight change as a predictor of child weight change in family-based behavioral obesity treatment. Arch Pediatr Adolesc Med. 2004;158:342–7.

Chapter 4 Understanding your child's weight

Barlow S and Dietz W. Obesity evaluation and treatment: Expert committee recommendations. Pediatrics. 1998;102(3). Accessed online April 14, 2005, at www.pediatrics.org/cgi/content/full/102/3/e29.

Centers for Disease Control and Prevention. BMI - Body Mass Index: BMI for Children and Teens. Accessed online May 4, 2005, at www.cdc.gov/nccdphp/dnpa/bmi/bmi-for-age.htm.

Daniels SR, Arnett DK, Eckel RH, Gidding SS, Hayman LL, Kumanyika S, Robinson TN, Scott BJ, St Jeor S, Williams CL. Overweight in children and adolescents: pathophysiology, consequences, prevention, and treatment. Circulation. 2005;111:1999–2012.

Epstein LH, Valoski AM, Kalarchian MA, McCurley J. Do children lose and maintain weight easier than adults: a comparison of child and parent weight changes from six months to ten years. Obes Res. 1995;3:411–7.

Epstein LH, Valoski A, Wing RR, McCurley J. Ten-year outcomes of behavioral family-based treatment for childhood obesity. Health Psychol. 1994;13:371–2.

Fowler-Brown, A., Kahwati, LC. Prevention and treatment of overweight in children and adolescents. Am Fam Physician. 2004;69:2591–8.

Kleinman RE, ed. Pediatric Nutrition Handbook, Fifth Edition. Chicago, IL: American Academy of Pediatrics, 2004.

Mueller WH. The changes with age of the anatomical distribution of fat. Soc Sci Med. 1982;16:191–6.

Must A, Jacques PF, Dallal GE, Bajema CJ, Dietz WH. Long-term morbidity and mortality of overweight adolescents: a follow-up of the Harvard Growth Study of 1922 to 1935. N Engl J Med. 1992;327:1350–5.

Narayan KM, Boyle JP, Thompson TJ, Sorensen SW, Williamson DF. Lifetime risk for diabetes mellitus in the United States. JAMA. 2003;290:1884–90.

National Task Force on the Prevention and Treatment of Obesity. Overweight, obesity, and health risk. Arch Intern Med. 2000;160:898–904.

Prevalence of Overweight among Children and Adolescents: United States, 1999–2002. Centers for Disease Control and Prevention, National Center for Health Statistics. Accessed online May 4, 2005, at www.cdc.gov/nchs/products/pubs/pubd/hestats/overwght99.htm.

Schwartz MB, Puhl R. Childhood obesity: a societal problem to solve. Obes Rev. 2003;4:57–71.

Williams CL, Strobino BA, Bollella M, Brotanek J. Cardiovascular risk reduction in preschool children: the "Healthy Start" project. J Am Coll Nutr. 2004;23:117–23.

Chapter 5 Changing your family's lifestyle

Prochaska JO, Velicer WF. The transtheoretical

model of health behavior change. *Am J Health Promot*. 1997;12:38–48.

Velicer WF, Rossi JS, Diclemente CC, Prochaska JO. A criterion measurement model for health behavior change. *Addict Behav*. 1996;21:555–84.

Chapter 6 How to get started

2005 Dietary Guidelines Advisory Committee Report. Accessed online August 8, 2005 at www.health.gov/dietaryguidelines/dga2005/report.

American Academy of Pediatrics. Policy Statement. Prevention of pediatric overweight and obesity. 2003;112:424–30. Accessed April 14, online at www.pediatrics.org.

Anderson RE, Crespo CJ, Bartlett SJ, Cheskin LJ, Pratt M. Relationship of physical activity and television watching with body weight and level of fatness among children: results from the Third National health and Nutrition Examination Survey. *JAMA*. 1998;279:938–42.

Berkey CS, Rockett HR, Gillman MW, Colditz GA. One-year changes in activity and in inactivity among 10- to 15-year-old boys and girls: relationship to change in body mass index. *Pediatrics*. 2003;111:836–43.

Biddle S, Sallis JF, Cavill NA. *Young and Active? Young People and Health Enhancing Physical Activity. Evidence and Implication*. London: Health Education Authority, 1998.

Birch LL, Davison KK. Family environmental factors influencing the developing behavioral controls of food intake and childhood overweight. *Pediatr Clin North Am*. 2001;48:893–907.

Bowman SA. Beverage choices of young females: changes and impact on nutrient intakes. *J Am Diet Assoc*. 2002;102:1234–9.

Cavill NA, Biddle S, Sallis JF. Health enhancing physical activity for young people: statement of the United Kingdom Expert Consensus Conference. *Pediatric Exercise Science*. 2001;13:12–25.

Clauss SB, Kwiterovich PO. Long-term safety and efficacy of low-fat diets in children and adolescents. *Minerva Pediatr*. 2002;54:305–13.

Deckelbaum RJ, Williams CL. Childhood obesity: the health issue. *Obes Res*. 2001;9:S239–43.

Dennison BA, Erb TA, Jenkins PL. Television viewing and television in bedroom associated with overweight risk among low-income preschool children. *Pediatrics*. 2002;109:1028–35.

Drewnowski A. Taste preferences and food intake. *Ann Rev Nutr*. 1997;17:237–53.

Edwards CA, Parrett AM. Dietary fibre in infancy and childhood. *Proc Nutr Soc*. 2003;62:17–23.

Field AE, Gillman MW, Rosner B, Rockett HR, Colditz GA. Associations between fruit and vegetable intake and change in body mass index among a large sample of children and adolescents in the United States. *Int J Obes*. 2003;27: 821–6.

Gillman MW, Rifas-Shiman SL, Frazier AL, Rockett HR, Camargo CA Jr, Field AE, Berkey CS, Colditz GA. Family dinner and diet quality among older children and adolescents. *Arch Fam Med*. 2000;9:235–40.

Golan M, Weizman A. Familial approach to the treatment of childhood obesity: conceptual mode. *J Nutr Educ*. 2001;33:102–7.

Hancox RJ, Milne BJ, Poulton R. Association between child and adolescent television viewing and adult health: a longitudinal birth cohort study. *Lancet*. 2004;364:257–62.

Harnack L, Stang J, Story M. Soft drink consumption among US children and adolescents: nutritional consequences. *J Am Diet Assoc*. 1999;99:436–41.

James J, Thomas P, Cavan D, Kerr D. Preventing childhood obesity by reducing consumption of carbonated drinks: cluster randomised controlled trial. *BMJ*. 2004;328:1237. Epub 2004 Apr 23.

Levin S, Lowry R, Brown DR, Dietz WH. Physical activity and body mass index among US adolescents. *Arch Pediatr Adolesc Med*. 2003;157:816–20.

Nicklas T, Johnson R; American Dietetic Association. Position of the American Dietetic Association: dietary guidance for healthy children ages 2 to 11 years. *J Am Diet Assoc*. 2004;104:660–77.

Orlet Fisher J, Rolls BJ, Birch LL. Children's bite size and intake of an entree are greater with large portions than with age-appropriate or self-selected portions. *Am J Clin Nutr*. 2003;77:1164–70.

Physical Activity and Health: A Report of the Surgeon General. Atlanta, GA: US Department of Health and Human Services, Centers for Disease Control and Prevention, National Center for Chronic Disease Prevention and Health Promotion, 1996.

Rajeshwari R, Yang SJ, Nicklas TA, Berenson GS. Secular trends in children's sweetened-beverage consumption (1973 to 1994): the Bogalusa Heart Study. *J Am Diet Assoc*. 2005;105:208–14.

Rampersaud GC, Pereira MA, Girard BL, Adams J, Metzl JD. Breakfast habits, nutritional status, body weight, and academic performance in children and adolescents. *J Am Diet Assoc*. 2005;105:743–60.

Ritchie LD, Welk G, Styne D, Gerstein DE, Crawford PB. Family environment and pediatric overweight: what is a parent to do? *J*

Am Diet Assoc. 2005;105:S70–9.

Rolls BJ, Engell D, Birch LL. Serving portion size influences 5-year-old but not 3-year-old children's food intakes. *J Am Diet Assoc.* 2000;100:232–4.

St-Onge MP, Keller KL, Heymsfield SB. Changes in childhood food consumption patterns: a cause for concern in light of increasing body weights. *Am J Clin Nutr* 2003;78:1068–73.

Williams CL, Hayman LL, Daniels SR, Robinson TN, Steinberger J, Paridon S, Bazzarre T. Cardiovascular health in childhood: a statement for health professionals from the Committee on Atherosclerosis, Hypertension, and Obesity in the Young (AHOY) of the Council on Cardiovascular Disease in the Young, American Heart Association. *Circulation.* 2002;106:143–60.

Wyatt HR, Grunwald GK, Mosca CL, Klem MI, Wing RR, Hill JO. Long-term weight loss and breakfast in subjects in the National Weight Control Registry. *Obes Res.* 2002;10:78–82.

Young LR, Nestle M. The contribution of expanding portion sizes to the US obesity epidemic. *Am J Public Health.* 2002;92:246–9.

Young LR, Nestle M. Expanding portion sizes in the US marketplace: implications for nutrition counseling. *J Am Diet Assoc.* 2003;103:231–4.

Chapter 7 The roles parents play;
Chapter 8 Putting the roles into action

Barlow SE, Dietz W, Jr Obesity evaluation and treatment: expert committee recommendations. *Pediatrics.*1998;102:e29.

Benton D. Role of parents in the determination of the food preferences of children and the development of obesity *Int J Relat Metab Disord.* 2004;28:858–69.

Birch LL, Davison KK. Family environmental

factors influencing the developing behavioral controls of food intake and childhood overweight. *Pediatric Clinics of North America.* 2001;48:893–907.

Birch LL, Deysher M. Caloric compensation and sensory specific satiety: evidence for self regulation of food intake by young children. *Appetite.*1986;7:323–31.

Birch LL, Fisher JO. Development of eating behaviors among children and adolescents. *Pediatrics.* 1998;101:539–49.

Birch LL, Marlin D, Rotter J. Eating as the "means" activity in a contingency: effects on young children's food preference. Child Dev. 1984;55:532–9.

Birch LL, Zimmerman S, Hind H. The influence of social affective context on preschool children's food preferences. *Child Dev.* 1980;51:856–61.

Birch LL. Generalization of a modified food preference. *Child Dev.* 1981;52:755–8.

Committee on Nutrition. Prevention of pediatric overweight and obesity. *Pediatrics.* 2003;112:424–30.

Cooke LJ, Wardle J, Gibson EL, Sapochnik M, Sheiham A, Lawson M. Demographic, familial and trait predictors of fruit and vegetable consumption by pre-school children. *Public Health Nutr.* 2004;7:295–302.

Coon KA, Goldberg J, Rogers BL, Tucker KL. Relationships between use of television during meals and children's food consumption patterns. *Pediatrics.* 2001;107:e7.

Cullen KW, Baranowski T, Owens E, Marsh T, Rittenberry L, de Moor C. Availability, accessibility, and preferences for fruit, 100% fruit juice, and vegetables influence children's dietary behavior. *Health Educ Behav.* 2003;30:615–26.

Ebbeling CB, Sinclair KB, Pereira MA,

Garcia-Lago E, Feldman HA, Ludwig DS. Compensation for energy intake from fast food among overweight and lean adolescents. *JAMA.* 2004;291:2828–33.

Eisenberg ME, Olson RE, Neumark-Sztainer D, Story M, Bearinger LH. Correlations between family meals and psychosocial well-being among adolescents. *Arch Pediatr Adolesc Med.* 2004;158:792–6.

Faddy eating: Dr Gillian Harris, consultant psychologist, Birmingham Children's Hospital and lecturer at Birmingham University. BBC Radio 4 Food Programme broadcast 10 Feb 2008.

Fisher JO, Birch LL. Restricting access to foods and children's eating. *Appetite.* 1999;32:405–19

Fox MK, Pac S, Devaney B, Jankowski L. Feeding infants and toddlers study: what foods are infants and toddlers eating? *J Am Diet Assoc.* 2004;104:S22–30.

Gillman MW, Rifas-Shiman SL, Frazier AL, Rockett HR, Camargo CA Jr, Field AE, Berkey CS, Colditz GA. Family dinner and diet quality among older children and adolescents. *Arch Fam Med.* 2000;9:235–40.

Golan M, Crow S. Targeting parents exclusively in the treatment of childhood obesity. long-term results. *Obes Res.* 2004;12:357–61.

Golan M, Weizman A, Apter A, Fainaru M. Parents as the exclusive agents of change in the treatment of childhood obesity. *Am J Clin Nutr.* 1998;67:1130–5.

Golan M, Weizman A. Familial approach to the treatment of childhood obesity: conceptual mode. *J Nutr Educ.* 2001;33:102–7.

Granner ML, Sargent RG, Calderon KS, Hussey JR, Evans AE, Watkins KW. Factors of fruit and vegetable intake by race, gender, and age among young adolescents. *J Nutr Educ Behav.* 2004;36:173–80.

Hanson NI, Neumark-Sztainer D, Eisenberg ME, Story M, Wall M. Associations between parental report of the home food environment and adolescent intakes of fruits, vegetables and dairy foods. *Public Health Nutr.* 2005;8:77–85.

Hood MY, Moore LL, Sundarajan-Ramamurti A, Singer M, Cupples LA, Ellison RC. Parental eating attitudes and the development of obesity in children. The Framingham Children's Study. *Int J Obes Relat Metab Disord.* 2000;24:1319–25.

Institute of Medicine of the National Academies. *Preventing Childhood Obesity: Health in the Balance.* Washington, DC: The National Academies Press, 2005.

Johnson SL, McPhee L, Birch LL. Conditioned preferences: young children prefer flavors associated with high dietary fat. *Physiol Behav.* 1991;50:1245–51.

Johnson SL. Improving preschoolers' self-regulation of energy intake. *Pediatrics.* 2000;106:1429–35.

Kremers SP, Bur J, De Vries H, Engels RC. Parenting style and adolescent fruit consumption. *Appetite.* 2003;42:43–50.

Lande B, Andersen LF, Veierod MB, Baerug A, Johansson L, Trygg KU, Bjorneboe GE. Breast-feeding at 12 months of age and dietary habits among breast-fed and non-breast-fed infants. *Public Health Nutr.* 2004;7:495–503.

Le Bigot Macaux A. Eat to live or live to eat? Do parents and children agree? *Public Health Nutr.* 2001;4:141–6.

Lederman SA, Akabas SR, Moore BJ, Bentley ME, Devaney B, Gillman MW, Kramer MS, Mennella JA, Ness A, Wardle J. Summary of the presentations at the Conference on Preventing Childhood Obesity, December 8, 2003. *Pediatrics.* 2004;114:1146–73.

Liem DG, Mars M, De Graaf C. Sweet preference and sugar consumption of 4- and 5-year-old children: role of parents. *Appetite.* 2004;43:235–45.

Loewen R, Pliner P. Effects of prior exposure to palatable and unpalatable novel foods on children's willingness to taste other novel foods. *Appetite.* 1999;32:351–66.

Ludwig DS, Peterson KE, Gortmaker SL. Relation between consumption of sugar-sweetened drinks and childhood obesity: a prospective, observational analysis. *Lancet.* 2001;357:505–8.

Marquis M, Filion YP, Dagenais F. Does eating while watching television influence children's food-related behaviours? *Can J Diet Pract Res.* 2005;66:12–8.

McCaffree J. Childhood eating patterns: the roles parents play. *J Am Diet Assoc.* 2003;103:1587.

McConahy KL, Smiciklas-Wright H, Birch LL, Mitchell DC, Picciano MF. Food portions are positively related to energy intake and body weight in early childhood. *J Pediatr.* 2002;140:340–7.

Neumark-Sztainer D, Wall M, Story M, Fulkerson JA. Are family meal patterns associated with disordered eating behaviors among adolescents? *J Adolesc Health.* 2004;35:350–9.

Nicklaus S, Boggio V, Chabanet C, Issanchou S. A prospective study of food variety seeking in childhood, adolescence and early adult life. *Appetite.* 2005;44:289–97.

Orlet Fisher J, Rolls BJ, Birch LL. Children's bite size and intake of an entree are greater with large portions than with age-appropriate or self-selected portions. *Am J Clin Nutr.* 2003;77:1164–70.

Pliner P, Loewen R. The effects of manipulated arousal on children's willingness to taste novel foods. *Physiol Behav.* 2002;76:551–8.

Roberts BP, Blinkhorn AS, Duxbury JT. The power of children over adults when obtaining sweet snacks. *Int J Paediatr Dent.* 2003;13:76–84.

Rolls BJ, Engell D, Birch LL. Serving portion size influences 5-year-old but not 3-year-old children's food intakes. *J Am Diet Assoc.* 2000;100:232–4.

Shunk JA, Birch LL. Girls at risk for overweight at age 5 are at risk for dietary restraint, disinhibited overeating, weight concerns, and great weight gain from 5 to 9 years. *J Am Diet Assoc.* 2004;104:1120–6.

Stice E, Presnell K, Shaw H, Rohde P. Psychological and behavioral risk factors for obesity onset in adolescent girls: a prospective study. *J Consult Clin Psychol.* 2005;73:195–202.

Story M, Holt K, Sofka D. *Bright Futures in Practice: Nutrition, 2nd ed.* Arlington, VA: National Center for Education in Maternal and Child Health, 2002.

Sullivan SA, Birch LL. Infant dietary experience and acceptance of solid foods. *Pediatrics.* 1994; 93:271-7.

Videon TM, Manning CK. Influences on adolescent eating patterns: the importance of family meals. *J Adolesc Health.* 2003;32:365–73.

Whitaker RC, Wright JA, Pepe MS, Seidel KD, Dietz WH. Predicting obesity in young adulthood from childhood and parental obesity. *N Engl J Med.* 1997;337:869–73

Chapter 9 Active parents, active children

2005 Dietary Guidelines Advisory Committee Report. Accessed online August 8, 2005 at www.health.gov/dietaryguidelines/dga2005/report/.

American Academy of Pediatrics Committee

on Public Education. Children, adolescents, and television. *Pediatrics.* 2001;107:423–6.

Anderssen N, Wold B. Parental and peer influences on leisure-time physical activity in young adolescents. *Res Q Exerc Sport.* 1992;63:341–8.

Arluk SL, Branch JD, Swain DP, Dowling EA. Childhood obesity's relationship to time spent in sedentary behavior. *Mil Med.* 2003;168:583–6.

Bandura A. Self-efficacy: the exercise of control *Am J Health Promotion.* 1997;12:8–12.

Barlow S, Dietz W. Obesity evaluation and treatment: expert committee recommendations. *Pediatrics.* 1998;102: e29. Accessed online April 14, 2005, at www. pediatrics.org/cgi/content/full/102/3/e29.

Baur LA, O'Connor J. Special considerations in childhood and adolescent obesity. *Clin Dermatol.* 2004;22:338–44

Biddle S, Goudas M. Analysis of children's physical activity and its association with adult encouragement and social cognitive values. *J School Health.* 1996;66:75–8.

Brustad RJ. Attraction to physical activity in urban schoolchildren: Parental socialization and gender influences. *Res Q Exerc Sport.* 1996;68:316–23.

Brustad RJ. Parental and peer influence on children's psychological development through sport. In Smoll FL, Smith RE (Eds.). *Children and Youth in Sport: A Biopsychosocial Perspective.* Madison, WI: Brown and Benchmark, 1996.

Brustad RJ. Who will go out and play? Parental and psychological influences on children's attraction to physical activity. *Pediatric Exercise Science.* 1993;5:210–23.

Chakravarthy MV, Booth FW. Inactivity and inaction. *Arch Pediatr Adolesc Med.*

2003;157:731–2.

Childwise Report on Children's TV and Internet Use, Jan 2008.

Craig S, Goldberg J, Dietz WH. Psychosocial correlates of physical activity among fifth and eighth graders. *Prev Med.* 1996;25:506–13.

Daniels SR, Arnett DK, Eckel RH, Gidding SS, Hayman LL, Kumanyika S, Robinson TN, Scott BJ, St Jeor S, Williams CL. Overweight in children and adolescents: pathophysiology, consequences, prevention, and treatment. *Circulation.* 2005;111:1999–2012.

Davison KK, Birch LL. Obesigenic families: parents' physical activity and dietary intake patterns predict girls' risk of overweight. *Int J Obes Relat Metab Disord.* 2002;26:1186–93.

Davison KK, Cutting TM, Birch LL. Parents' activity-related parenting practices predict girls' physical activity. *Med Sci Sports Exerc.* 2003;35:1589–95.

Dennison BA, Erb TA, Jenkins PL. Television viewing and television in bedroom associated with overweight risk among low-income preschool children. *Pediatrics.* 2002;109:1028–35.

DiLorenzo TM, Stucky-Ropp RC, Vander Wal JS, Gotham HJ. Determinants of exercise among children. II. A longitudinal analysis. *Prev Med.* 1998;27:470–7

Epstein LH, Paluch RA, Gordy CC, Dorn J. Decreasing sedentary behaviors in treating pediatric obesity. *Arch Pediatr Adolesc Med.* 2000;154:220–6.

Epstein LH, Valoski AM, Vara LS, McCurley J, Wisniewski L, Kalarchian MA, Klein KR, Shrager LF. Effects of decreasing sedentary behavior and increasing activity on weight change in obese children. *Health Psychol.* 1995;14:109–15.

Faith MS, Leone MA, Ayers TS, Heo M,

Pietrobelli A. Weight criticism during physical activity, coping skills, and reported physical activity in children. *Pediatrics.* 2002;110:e23.

Fogelholm M, Nuutinen O, Pasanen M, Myohanen E, Saatela T. Parent-child relationship of physical activity patterns and obesity. *Int J Obes Relat Metab Disord.* 1999;23:1262–8.

Fowler-Brown A, Kahwati LC. Prevention and treatment of overweight in children and adolescents. *Am Fam Physician.* 2004;69:2591–8.

Freedson PS, Evenson S. Familial aggregation in physical activity. *Res Q Exerc Sport.* 1991;62:384–9.

Golan M, Fainaru M, Weizman A. Role of behaviour modification in the treatment of childhood obesity with the parents as the exclusive agents of change. *Int J Obes Relat Metab Disord.* 1998;22:1217–24.

Golan M, Weizman A. Familial approach to the treatment of childhood obesity: conceptual mode. *J Nutr Educ.* 2001;33:102–7.

Gortmaker SL, Must A, Sobol AM, Peterson K, Colditz GA, Dietz WH. Television viewing as a cause of increasing obesity among children in the United States, 1986–1990. *Arch Pediatr Adolesc Med.* 1996;150:356–62.

Gutin B, Yin Z, Humphries MC, Barbeau P. Relations of moderate and vigorous physical activity to fitness and fatness in adolescents. *Am J Clin Nutr.* 2005;81:746–50.

Health Survey for England 1994-2003. Department of Health.

Healthy People 2010. Accessed online May 11, 2005, at www.healthypeople.gov.

Healthy Weight, Healthy Lives. Department of Health 2008.

Institute of Medicine of the National

references and sources

Academies. *Preventing Childhood Obesity, Health in the Balance.* Washington, DC: The National Academies Press, 2005.

Kalakanis LE, Goldfield GS, Paluch RA, Epstein LH. Parental activity as a determinant of activity level and patterns of activity in obese children. *Res Q Exerc Sport.* 2001;72:202–9.

Kimiecik JC, Horn TS, Shurin CS. Relationships among children's beliefs, perceptions of their parents' beliefs, and their moderate-to-vigorous physical activity. *Res Q Exer Sport.* 1966;67:324–36.

Kimiecik JC, Horn TS. Parental beliefs and children's moderate-to-vigorous physical activity. *Res Q Exerc Sport.* 1998;69:163–75.

Kohl HW, Hobbs KE. Development of physical activity behaviors among children and adolescents. *Pediatrics* 1998;101:549–54

McGuire MT, Hannan PJ, Neumark-Sztainer D, Cossrow NH, Story M. Parental correlates of physical activity in a racially/ethnically diverse adolescent sample. *J Adolesc Health.* 2002;30:253–61.

McKenzie TL, Li D, Derby CA, Webber LS, Luepker RV, Cribb P. Maintenance of effects of the CATCH physical education program: results from the CATCH-ON study. *Health Educ Behav.* 2003;30:447–62.

Moore LL, Lombardi DA, White MJ, Campbell JL, Oliveria SA, Ellison RC. Influence of parents' physical activity levels on activity levels of young children. *J Pediatr.* 1991;118:215–9.

Patrick K, Spear B, Holt K, Sofka D, eds. Bright Futures in Practice: Physical Activity. Arlington, VA: National Center for Education in Maternal and Child Health, 2001.

Perez CE. Children who become active. *Health Rep.* 2003;14 (Suppl:) 17–28.

Proctor MH, Moore LL, Gao D, Cupples LA, Bradlee ML, Hood MY, Ellison RC. Television viewing and change in body fat from preschool to early adolescence: the Framingham Children's Study. *Int J Obes Relat Disord.* 2003;27:827–33.

Ritchie LD, Welk G, Styne D, Gerstein DE, Crawford PB. Family environment and pediatric overweight: what is a parent to do? *J Am Diet Assoc.* 2005;105:S70–9.

Robinson TN, Killen JD, Kraemer HC, Wilson DM, Matheson DM, Haskell WL, Pruitt LA, Powell TM, Owens AS, Thompson NS, Flint-Moore NM, Davis GJ, Emig KA, Brown RT, Rochon J, Green S, Varady A. Dance and reducing television viewing to prevent weight gain in African-American girls: the Stanford GEMS pilot study. *Ethn Dis.* 2003;13:S65–77.

Sallis JF, McKenzie TL, Elder JP, Broyles SL, Nader PR. Factors parents use in selecting play spaces for young children. *Arch Pediar Adolesc Med.* 1997;151:414–7.

Sallis JF, Prochaska JJ, Taylor WC. A review of correlates of physical activity of children and adolescents. *Med Sci Sports Exerc.* 2000;32:963–75.

Scanlan TK, Simons JP. The construct of sports enjoyment. In GC Roberts (Ed.), *Motivation in Sport and Exercise.* Champaign, IL: *Human Kinetics,* 1992.

Shape Up America! Accessed online May 24, 2005, at www.shapeupamerica.org.

Statistics on obesity, physical activity and diet. England 2006, NHS.

Stucky-Ropp RC, DiLorenzo TM. Determinants of exercise in children. *Prev Med.* 1993;22:880–9.

Trost SG, Pate RR, Saunders R, Ward DS, Dowda M, Felton G. A prospective study of the determinants of physical activity in rural fifth-grade children. *Prev Med.* 1997;26:257–63.

Trost SG, Sallis JF, Pate RR, Freedson PS,

Taylor WC, Dowda M. Evaluating a model of parental influence on youth physical activity. *Am J Prev Med.* 2003;25:277–82.

Trost SG, Sirard JR, Dowda M, Pfeiffer KA, Pate RR. Physical activity in overweight and nonoverweight preschool children. *Int J Obes Relat Metab Disord.* 2003;27:834–9.

U.S. Surgeon General. *The Surgeon General's Call to Action to Prevent and Decrease Overweight and Obesity.* Accessed online August 8, 2005 at www.surgeongeneral.gov/topics/obesity/calltoaction/.

Wagner A, Klein-Platat C, Arveiler D, Haan MC, Schlienger JL, Simon C. Parent-child physical activity relationships in 12-year old French students do not depend on family socioeconomic status. *Diabetes Metab.* 2004;30:359–66.

Weight-control Information Network. Accessed online May 11, 2005, at http://win.niddk.nih.gov/index.htm.

Welk, GJ. *Promoting Physical Activity in Children: Parental Influences.* Washington, DC: ERIC Clearinghouse on Teaching and Teacher Education, 2000. Accessed online on May 11, 2005 at www.ericdigests.org/2000-3/activity.htm.

Welk GJ. *Promoting Physical Activity in Children: Parental Influences.* Washington DC: ERIC Clearinghouse on Teaching and Teacher Education, 1999.

Weiss MR, Ebbeck V. Self-esteem and perceptions of competence in youth sport: theory, research, and enhancement strategies. In Bar-Or O (Ed.). *The Encyclopedia of Sports Medicine, Volume 4: The Child and Adolescent Athlete.* Oxford UK: Blackwell Science 1996.

Weiss MR. Motivating kids in physical activity. *President's Council on Physical Fitness and Sports Research Digest.* Series 3, No. 11, September 2000.

Welsh Health Survey 2003/4. National Assembly for Wales.

Whitaker RC. Obesity prevention in pediatric primary care. *Arch Pediatr Adolesc Med.* 2003;157:725–7.

Writing Group. Understanding obesity in youth. *Circulation.* 1996;94:3383–87.

Chapter 10 Looking after your children

Bell SK, Morgan SB. Children's attitudes and behavioral intentions toward a peer presented as obese: does a medical explanation for the obesity make a difference? *J Pediatr Psychol.* 2000;25:137–145.

Braet C, Mervielde I, Vandereycken W. Psychological aspects of childhood obesity: a controlled study in a clinical and nonclinical sample. *J Pediatr Psychol.* 1997;22:59–71.

Brehm BJ, Rourke KM, Cassell C, Sethuraman G. Psychosocial outcomes of a pilot multidisciplinary program for weight management. *Am J Health Behav.* 2003;27:348–54.

Family pediatrics: report of the Task Force on the Family. *Pediatrics.* 2003;111:1541–71.

Janssen I, Craig WM, Boyce WF, Pickett W. Associations between overweight and obesity with bullying behaviors in school-aged children. *Pediatrics.* 2004;113:1187–94.

Kramer L, Perozynski LA, Chung TY. Parental responses to sibling conflict: the effects of development and parent gender. *Child Dev.* 1999;70:1401–14.

Latner JD, Stunkard AJ. Getting worse: the stigmatization of obese children. *Obes Res.* 2003;11:452–6.

Malina RM. Physical activity and fitness: pathways from childhood to adulthood. *Am J Hum Biol.* 2001;13:162–72.

Malina RM. Tracking of physical activity and physical fitness across the lifespan. *Res Q Exerc Sport.* 1996;67:S548–57.

Manus HE, Killeen MR. Maintenance of self-esteem by obese children. *J Child Adolesc Psychiatr Nurs.* 1995;8:17–27.

Marinov B, Kostianev S, Turnovska T. Ventilatory efficiency and rate of perceived exertion in obese and non-obese children performing standardized exercise. *Clin Physiol Funct Imaging.* 2002;22:254–60.

Musher-Eizenman DR, Holub SC, Miller AB, Goldstein SE, Edwards-Leeper L. Body size stigmatization in preschool children: the role of control attributions. *J Pediatr Psychol.* 2004;29:613–20.

Neumark-Sztainer D, Story M, Hannan PJ, Tharp T, Rex J. Factors associated with changes in physical activity: a cohort study of inactive adolescent girls. *Arch Pediatr Adolesc Med.* 2003;157.803–10.

Norman A-C, Drinkard B, McDuffie JR, Ghorbani S, Yanoff YB, Yanovski JA. Influence of excess adiposity on exercise fitness and performance in overweight children and adolescents. *Pediatrics.* 2005;115:e690.

Robbins LB, Pender NJ, Kazanis AS. Barriers to physical activity perceived by adolescent girls. *J Midwifery Womens Health.* 2003;48:203–12.

Schor EL. Developing communality: family-centered programs to improve children's health and well-being. *Bull NY Acad Med.* 1995;72:413–42.

Strauss RS. Childhood obesity and self-esteem. *Pediatrics.* 2000;105:e15.

Strauss RS, Pollack HA. Social marginalization of overweight children. *Arch Pediatr Adolsc Med.* 2003;157:746–52.

Taylor WC, Yancey AK, Leslie J, Murray NG,

Cummings SS, Sharkey SA, Wert C, James J, Miles O, McCarthy WJ. Physical activity among African American and Latino middle school girls: consistent beliefs, expectations, and experiences access two sites. *Women Health.* 1999;30:67–82.

Timm NL, Grupp-Phelan J, Ho ML. Chronic ankle morbidity in obese children following an acute ankle injury. *Arch Pediatr Adolesc Med.* 2005;159.33–6.

Zabinski MF, Saelens BE, Stein RI, Hayden-Wade HA, Wilfley DE. Overweight children's barriers to and support for physical activity. *Obes Res.* 2003;11:238–46.

Chapter 11 Taking the message outside the home

Barlow SE, Dietz, WH. Obesity evaluation and treatment: expert committee recommendations. *Pediatrics.* 1998;102:e29.

Batch JA, Baur LA. Management and prevention of obesity and its complications in children and adolescents. *Med J Aust.* 2005;182:130–5.

Borra ST, Kelly L, Shirreffs MB, Neville K, Geiger CJ. Developing health messages: qualitative studies with children, parents, and teachers help identify communications opportunities for healthful lifestyles and the prevention of obesity. *J Am Diet Assoc.* 2003;103:721–8.

Caballero B. Obesity prevention in children: opportunitites and challenges. *Int J Obes Relat Metab Disord.* 2004;28:S90–5.

Carlisle LK, Gordon ST, Sothern MS. Can obesity prevention work for our children? *J La State Med Soc.* 2005;157:S34–41.

Children's Dental Health Survey, Office National Statistics 2003.

Dietz WH, Gortmaker SL. Preventing obesity in children and adolescents. *Annu Rev Public Health.* 2001;22:337–53.

Dietz WH, Robinson TN. Overweight children and adolescents. *N Engl J Med* 2005;352:2100–9.

Institute of Medicine of the National Academies. *Preventing Childhood Obesity, Health in the Balance.* Washington, D.C.: The National Academies Press, 2005.

Lissau I, Sorensen TI. Parental neglect during childhood and increased risk of obesity in young adulthood. *Lancet.* 1994;343:324–7.

Lissau I, Sorensen TI. School difficulties in childhood and risk of overweight and obesity in young adulthood: a ten year prospective population study. *Int J Obes Relat Metab Disord.* 1993;17:169–75.

McCaffree J. Childhood eating patterns: the roles parents play. *J Am Diet Assoc.* 2003;103:1587.

Muller MJ, Asbeck I, Mast M, Langnase K, Grund A. Prevention of obesity—more than an intention. Concept and first results of the Kiel Obesity Prevention Study (KOPS). *Int J Obes Relat Metab Disord.* 2001;25:S66–74.

National Diet and Nutritional Survey, 4-18 years, 2000. Food Standards Agency

Olson CM. Childhood nutrition education in health promotion and disease prevention. *Bull NY Acad Med.* 1989;65:1143–53.

Shephard RJ. Role of the physician in childhood obesity. *Clin J Sport Med.* 2004;14:161–8.

Williams CL. Nutrition intervention and health risk reduction in childhood: creating healthy adults. *Pediatrician.* 1983-85;12:97–101.

Chapter 12 Different families have different needs

Adams RA, Gordon C, Spangler AA. Maternal stress in caring for children with feeding disabilities: implications for health care providers. *J Am Diet Assoc.* 1999;99:962–6.

Ayyangar R. Healthy maintenance and management in childhood disability. *Phys Med Rehabil Clin N Am.* 2002;13:793–821.

Baumrind D. Effects of authoritative control on child behavior. *Child Dev.* 1966;37:887–907.

Case-Smith J. Parenting a child with a chronic medical condition. *Am J Occup Ther.* 2004;58:551–60.

Crawford PB, Gosliner W, Anderson C Strode P, Becerra-Jones Y, Samuel S, Carroll AM, Ritchie LD. Counseling Latina mothers of preschool children about weight issues: suggestions for a new framework. *J Am Diet Assoc.* 2004;104:387–94.

Cummings EM, Goeke-Morey MC, Papp LM, Dukewich TL. Children's responses to mothers' and fathers' emotionality and tactics in marital conflict in the home. *J Fam Psychol.* 2002;16:478–92.

Eisenberg ME, Olson RE, Neumark-Sztainer D, Story M, Bearinger LH. Correlations between family meals and psychosocial well-being among adolescents. *Arch Pediatr Adolesc Med.* 2004;158:792–6.

Elder JH, Valcante G, Yarandi H, White D, Elder TH. Evaluating in-home training for fathers of children with autism using single-subject experimentation and group analysis methods. *Nurs Res.* 2005;54:22–32.

Family pediatrics report of the Task Force on the Family. *Pediatrics.* 2003;111:1541–71.

Federal Interagency Forum on Child and Family Statistics. *America's Children: Key national Indicators of Well-Being.* Washington, DC: US Government Printing Office; 1999.

Ford-Gilboe M. Family strengths, motivation, and resources as predictors of health promotion behavior in single-parent and two-parent families. *Res Nurs Health.* 1997;20:205–17.

Gillman MW, Rifas-Shiman SL, Frazier AL, Rockett HR, Carmargo CA Jr, Field AE, Berkey CS, Colditz GA. Family dinner and diet quality among older children and adolescents. *Arch Fam Med.* 2000;9:235–40.

Green SE. "What do you mean 'what's wrong with her?'": stigma and the lives of families of children with disabilities. *Soc Sci Med.* 2003;57:1361–74.

Kelly JB. Marital conflict, divorce, and children's adjustment. *Child Adolesc Psychiatr Clin N Am.* 1998;7:259–71.

Lobato DJ, Kao BT. Integrated sibling-parent group intervention to improve sibling knowledge and adjustment to chronic illness and disability. *J Pediatr Psychol.* 2002;27:711–6.

McLanahan S, Sandfur G. *Growing up with a single Parent: What Hurts, What Helps.* Cambridge, MA: Harvard University Press, 1994.

ONS Divorces: Couples and children of divorced couples, 1981, 1991, 2001-2005. Population Trends 125. Office for National Statistics.

Patrick H, Nicklas TA, Hughes SO, Morales M. The benefits of authoritative feeding style: caregiver feeding styles and children's food consumption patterns. *Appetite.* 2005;44:243–9.

Rippe JM, Price JM, Hess SA, Kline G, DeMers KA, Damitz S, Kreidieh I, Freedson P. Improved psychological well-being, quality of life, and health practices in moderately overweight women participating in a 12-week structured weight loss program. *Obes Res.* 1998;6:208-18.

Ritchie LD, Welk G, Styne D, Gerstein DE, Crawford PB. Family environment and pediatric overweight: what is a parent to do? *J Am Diet Assoc.* 2005;105:S70–9.

Shunk JA, Birch LL. Validity of dietary restraint among 5- to 9-year-old girls. *Appetite.* 2004;42:241–7.

Simons RL, Lin K-H, Gordon LC, Conger RD, Lorenz FO. Explaining the higher incidence of adjustment problems among children of divorce compared with those in two-parent families. *J Marriage Fam.* 1999;61:1020–33.

Spieker SJ, Larson NC, Lewis SM, Keller TE, Gilcrist L. Developmental trajectories of disruptive behavior problems in preschool children of adolescent mothers. *Child Dev.* 1999;70:443–58.

Troxel WM, Matthews KA. What are the costs of marital conflict and dissolution of children's physical health? *Clin Child Fam Psychol Rev.* 2004;7:29–57.

Videon TM, Manning CK. Influences on adolescent eating patterns: the importance of family meals. *J Adolesc Health.* 2003;32:365–73.

Williams PD, Williams AR, Graff JC, Hanson S, Stanton A, Hafeman C, Liebergen A, Leuenberg K, Setter RK, Ridder L, Curry H, Barnard M, Sanders S. Interrelationships among variables affecting well siblings and mothers in families of children with a chronic illness or disability. *J Behav Med.* 2002;25:411–24.

Chapter 13 Getting extra help

Atkinson RL, Nitzke SA. School-based progs on obesity. *BMJ.* 2001;323:1018–9.

Austin SB, Field AE, Wiecha J, Peterson KE, Gortmaker SL. The impact of a school-based obesity prevention trial on disordered weight-control behaviors in early adolescent girls. *Arch Pediatr Adolesc Med.* 2005;159:225–30.

Berkowitz RK, Wadden TA, Tershakovec AM, Cronquist JL. Behavior therapy and sibutramine for the treatment of adolescent obesity: a randomized clinical trial. *JAMA.* 2003;289:1805–12.

Bray GA. Drug treatment of obesity. *Rev Endocr Metab Disord.* 2001;2:403–18.

Bray GA, Blackburn GL, Ferguson JM, Greenway FL, Jain AK, Mendel CM, Mendels J, Ryan DH, Schwartz SL, Scheinbaum ML, Seaton TB. Sibutramine produces dose-related weight loss. *Obes Res.* 1999;7:189–98.

Chanoine JP, Hampl S, Jensen C, Boldrin M, Hauptman J. Effect of orlistat on weight and body composition in obese adolescents: a randomized controlled trial. *JAMA.* 2005;293:2873–83.

Daniels SR, Arnett DK, Eckel RH, Gidding SS, Hayman LL, Kumanyika S, Robinson TN, Scott BJ, St. Jeor S, Williams CL. Overweight in children and adolescents: pathophysiology, consequences, prevention, and treatment. *Circulation.* 2005;111:1999–2012.

Davidson MH, Hauptman J, DiGirolamo M, Foreyt JP, Halsted CH, Hebor D, Heimburger DC, Lucas CP, Robbins DC, Chung J, Heymsfield SB. Weight control and risk factor reduction in obese subjects treated for 2 years with orlistat: a randomized controlled trial. *JAMA.* 1999;281:235–42.

Flodmark C-E, Lissau I, Moreno LA, Pietrobelli A, Widhalm K. New insights into the field of children and adolescents' obesity. *Int J Obes.* 2004;28:1189–96.

Fowler-Brown A, Kahwati L. Prevention and treatment of overweight in children and adolescents. *Am Fam Physician.* 2004;69:2591–8.

Inge TH, Lawson L. Treatment considerations for severe adolescent obesity. *Surg Obes Rel Dis.* 2005;1:133–9.

Institute of Medicine. *Weighing the Options: Criteria for Evaluating Weight-Management Programs.* Washington, DC: National Academy Press, 1995.

Institute of Medicine of the National Academies. *Preventing Childhood Obesity: Health in the Balance.* Washington, DC: The National Academies Press, 2005.

Kirk S, Scott B, Daniels S. Pediatric obesity epidemic: treatment options. *J Am Diet Assoc.* 2005;105:S44–51.

Lumeng JC, Gannon K, Appugliese D, Cabral HJ, Zuckerman B. Preschool child care and risk of overweight in 6- to 12-year-old children. *Int J Obes Relat Metab Disord.* 2005;29:60–6.

McDuffe JR, Calis KA, Booth SL, Uwaifo GI, Yanovski JA. Effects of orlistat on fat soluble vitamins in obese adolescents. *Pharmacotherapy.* 2002;22:814–82?

Müller MJ, Asbeck I, Mast M, Langnase K, Grund A. Prevention of obesity—more than an intention: concept and first results of the Kiel Obesity Prevention Study (KOPS). *Int J Obes Relat Metab Disord.* 2001.;25:S66–74.

Pate RR, Trost SG, Mullis R, Sallis JF, Wechsler H, Brown DR. Community interventions to promote proper nutrition and physical activity among youth. *Prev Med.* 2000;31:S138–48.

Veugelers PJ, Fitzgerald AL. Effectiveness of school programs in preventing childhood obesity: a multilevel comparison. *Am J Public Health.* 2005;95:432–5.

Yin Z, Hanes J Jr, Moore JB, Humbles P, Barbeau P, Gutin B. An after-school physical activity program for obesity prevention in children: the Medical College of Georgia FitKid Project. *Eval Health Prof.* 2005;28:67–89.

index

index

E

eating disorders 43, 63, 153
energy balance 28
enforcer, being an 23

F

family meals, importance of 62, 83, 88, 93, 94, 97, 145, 146

food enforcer
    definition 77
    for babies 84
    for younger children 91
    for older children 97

food labels 96

food provider
    definition 75
    for babies 84
    for younger children 88
    for older children 96

food role model
    definition 74
    for babies 82
    for young children 86
    for older children 94

fruit juice 66, 67, 79
fussy eaters 84, 86

G

GPs 40, 42, 152, 153

H

genes 28

healthy-weight home 17
healthy-weight protector 126
hunger 76, 84, 87, 89, 97

N

nutritionist 152

O

obesity
    definition 41
    in adults 14, 42
    in children 14, 15, 42

older children
    activity enforcer for 120
    activity provider for 119
    activity role model for 118
    food enforcer for 97
    food provider for 96
    food role model for 94

online help 155

overweight
    definition 41
    at risk of 41

acknowledgements

picture credits

Front cover images, clockwise from top left: Roberta Parkin, Francine Lawrence, Photolibrary, Roberta Parkin, Photolibrary. Back cover images, from left to right: Mayan McKenzie, Jason Smalley, Roberta Parkin

All other images throughout the book from iStockphoto except where indicated below

Contents pp 8, 9
Clockwise from top left: Francine Lawrence, Roberta Parkin, Photolibrary, iStockphoto, Weight Watchers

Chapter 1
pp 13, 14 Photolibrary

Chapter 2
p22 Photolibrary

Chapter 3
p27 Photolibrary
p29 apple photo by Mayan McKenzie

Case study 1
p37 Jason Smalley

Chapter 4
p39 Photolibrary

Case study 2
p47 Francine Lawrence

Chapter 5
p50 Mikey Georgeson

Chapter 6
p59 Roberta Parkin
pp60, 61 Clockwise from top: Roberta Parkin, iStockphoto, Photolibrary, iStockphoto, Roberta Parkin

p63 Mayan McKenzie

p65 Roberta Parkin

Case study 3
p69 Francine Lawrence

Chapter 7
p73 Getty Images

Chapter 8
pp 91, 92, 95, 96, 99 Photolibrary

Chapter 9
p115 Photolibrary
p119 Roberta Parkin

Chapter 10
p124 Mayan McKenzie

Chapter 11
pp133, 139 Roberta Parkin
pp136, 137 Francine Lawrence

Chapter 13
p154 Photolibrary

Chapter 14
p159 Photolibrary
p161 Top to bottom: iStockphoto, Roberta Parkin, iStockphoto

pp162-181 All recipe pictures from Weight Watchers

Chapter 15
p185 Photolibrary

And thanks to:
Terry Barber and Jude Evans for proof-reading.
The kitchen staff and pupils of The Downs CE Primary School, Walmer, Kent

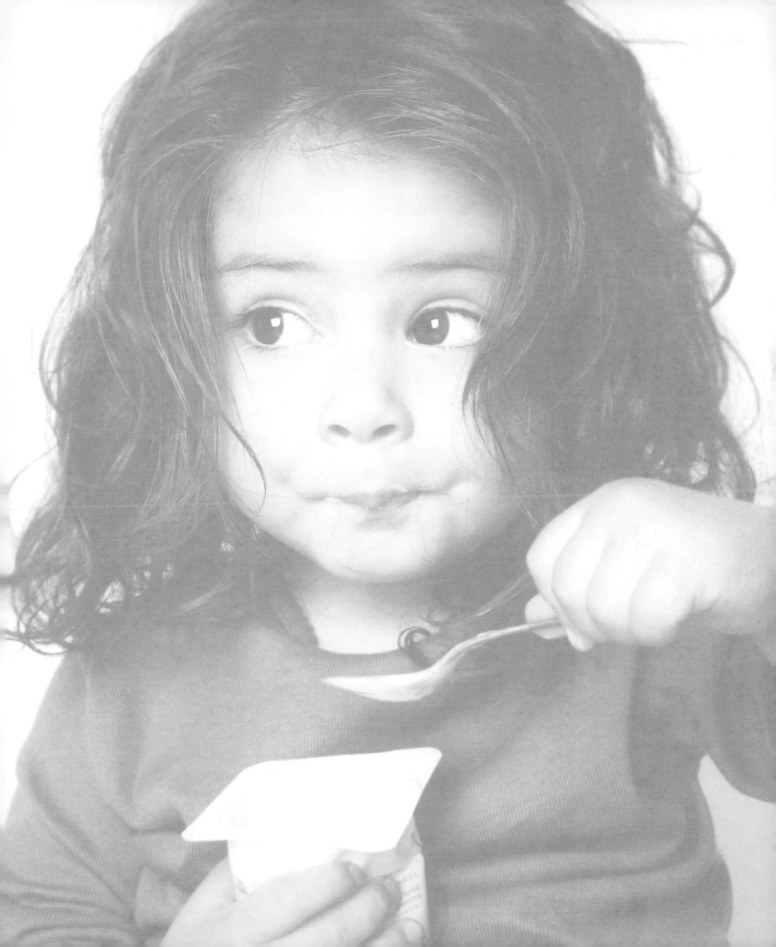